Ethnically Sensitive Rhinoplasty

Editors

ANTHONY E. BRISSETT
LISA E. ISHII
KOFI D.O. BOAHENE

OTOLARYNGOLOGIC CLINICS OF NORTH AMERICA

www.oto.theclinics.com

Consulting Editor
SUJANA S. CHANDRASEKHAR

April 2020 • Volume 53 • Number 2

ELSEVIER

1600 John F. Kennedy Boulevard • Suite 1800 • Philadelphia, Pennsylvania, 19103-2899

http://www.oto.theclinics.com

OTOLARYNGOLOGIC CLINICS OF NORTH AMERICA Volume 53, Number 2
April 2020 ISSN 0030-6665, ISBN-13: 978-0-323-71279-8

Editor: Stacy Eastman
Developmental Editor: Laura Fisher

Otolaryngologic Clinics of North America (ISSN 0030-6665) is published bimonthly by Elsevier, Inc., 360 Park Avenue South, New York, NY 10010-1710. Months of issue are February, April, June, August, October, and December. Business and Editorial Offices: 1600 John F. Kennedy Blvd., Suite 1800, Philadelphia, PA 19103-2899. Customer Service Office: 6277 Sea Harbor Drive, Orlando, FL 32887-4800. Periodicals postage paid at New York, NY and additional mailing offices. Subscription prices are $424.00 per year (US individuals), $947.00 per year (US institutions), $100.00 per year (US & Canadian student/resident), $548.00 per year (Canadian individuals), $1200.00 per year (Canadian institutions), $592.00 per year (international individuals), $1200.00 per year (international institutions), $270.00 per year (international student/resident). Foreign air speed delivery is included in all *Clinics'* subscription prices. All prices are subject to change without notice. **POSTMASTER:** Send address changes to *Otolaryngologic Clinics of North America*, Elsevier Health Sciences Division, Subscription Customer Service, 3251 Riverport Lane, Maryland Heights, MO 63043. **Telephone: 1-800-654-2452 (U.S. and Canada); 314-447-8871 (outside U.S. and Canada). Fax: 314-447-8029. E-mail: journalscustomerservice-usa@elsevier.com (for print support); journalsonlinesupport-usa@elsevier.com (for online support):**

Reprints. For copies of 100 or more of articles in this publication, please contact the Commercial Reprints Department, Elsevier Inc., 360 Park Avenue South, New York, NY 10010-1710. Tel.: 212-633-3874; Fax: 212-633-3820; E-mail: reprints@elsevier.com.

Otolaryngologic Clinics of North America is also published in Spanish by McGraw-Hill Interamericana Editores S.A., P.O. Box 5-237, 06500 Mexico D.F., Mexico.

Otolaryngologic Clinics of North America is covered in *MEDLINE/PubMed (Index Medicus), Current Contents/Clinical Medicine, Excerpta Medica, BIOSIS, Science Citation Index,* and *ISI/BIOMED.*

Contributors

CONSULTING EDITOR

SUJANA S. CHANDRASEKHAR, MD, FACS, FAAOHNS
Past President, American Academy of Otolaryngology–Head and Neck Surgery, Secretary-Treasurer, American Otological Society, Partner, ENT & Allergy Associates, LLP, Clinical Professor, Department of Otolaryngology–Head and Neck Surgery, Zucker School of Medicine at Hofstra-Northwell, Hempstead, New York, USA; Clinical Associate Professor, Department of Otolaryngology–Head and Neck Surgery, Icahn School of Medicine at Mount Sinai, New York, New York, USA

EDITORS

ANTHONY E. BRISSETT, MD, FACS
Vice Chair, Department Otolaryngology/Head and Neck Surgery, Division Chief, Division of Facial Plastic and Reconstructive Surgery, Adjunct Associate Professor, Texas A&M University College of Medicine, Houston Methodist ENT Specialists, Houston, Texas, USA

LISA E. ISHII, MD, MHS
Professor, Department of Otolaryngology–Head and Neck Surgery, The Johns Hopkins University School of Medicine, Johns Hopkins Outpatient Center, Baltimore, Maryland, USA

KOFI D.O. BOAHENE, MD, FACS
Professor, Otolaryngology Head and Neck Surgery, Division of Facial Plastic and Reconstructive Surgery, Department of Otolaryngology–Head and Neck Surgery, The Johns Hopkins University School of Medicine, Johns Hopkins Outpatient Center, Baltimore, Maryland, USA

AUTHORS

KOFI D.O. BOAHENE, MD, FACS
Professor, Otolaryngology Head and Neck Surgery, Division of Facial Plastic and Reconstructive Surgery, Department of Otolaryngology–Head and Neck Surgery, The Johns Hopkins University School of Medicine, Johns Hopkins Outpatient Center, Baltimore, Maryland, USA

ANTHONY E. BRISSETT, MD, FACS
Vice Chair, Department Otolaryngology/Head and Neck Surgery, Division Chief, Division of Facial Plastic and Reconstructive Surgery, Adjunct Associate Professor, Texas A&M University College of Medicine, Houston Methodist ENT Specialists, Houston, Texas, USA

ROXANA COBO, MD
Chief, Department of Otolaryngology, Centro Médico Imbanaco, Cali, Colombia

ROBERT DEEB, MD
Director, Division of Facial Plastic and Reconstructive Surgery, Department of Otolaryngology–Head and Neck Surgery, Henry Ford Health System, Henry Ford Hospital, Clinical Assistant Professor, Wayne State University School of Medicine, Detroit, Michigan, USA

HOLGER G. GASSNER, MD
Director, Finesse Center for Facial Plastic Surgery Regensburg, Clinical Professor, Faculty of Medicine, University of Regensburg, Regensburg, Germany

KATHERINE ELIZABETH HICKS, MD
Facial Plastic Surgery Fellow, Department of Otolaryngology–Head and Neck Surgery, Northwestern University, Chicago, Illinois, USA

LISA E. ISHII, MD, MHS
Professor, Department of Otolaryngology–Head and Neck Surgery, The Johns Hopkins University School of Medicine, Johns Hopkins Outpatient Center, Baltimore, Maryland, USA

YONG JU JANG, MD, PhD
Professor, Department of Otolaryngology, Asan Medical Center, University of Ulsan College of Medicine, Seoul, South Korea

ANISHA R. KUMAR, MD
Department of Otolaryngology–Head and Neck Surgery, Johns Hopkins School of Medicine, Johns Hopkins Outpatient Center, Johns Hopkins University, Baltimore, Maryland, USA

SAM P. MOST, MD
Division of Facial Plastic and Reconstructive Surgery, Stanford University School of Medicine, Stanford, California, USA

HYUNG GYUN NA, MD
Assistant Professor, Department of Otorhinolaryngology–Head and Neck Surgery, University of Yeungnam College of Medicine, Daegu, Korea

KATE O'CONNOR, MD
Houston Methodist Hospital, Baylor College of Medicine, Houston, Texas, USA

PRIYESH N. PATEL, MD
Division of Facial Plastic and Reconstructive Surgery, Stanford University School of Medicine, Stanford, California, USA

DAVID A. SHERRIS, MD
Professor and Chairman, Department of Otolaryngology, Jacobs School of Medicine and Biomedical Sciences, Buffalo, New York, USA

JAMES REGAN THOMAS, MD, FACS
Professor, Facial Plastic and Reconstructive Surgery, Department of Otolaryngology–Head and Neck Surgery, Northwestern School of Medicine, Chicago, Illinois, USA

Contents

Beauty is difficult to define. The US population becomes more diverse by the day. Thus, traditional stereotypes of beauty in various ethnic groups become less applicable as diversity increases. Often, new and uniquely beautiful facial features and proportions emerge as different ethnicities converge. With the increased diversity in facial appearance comes increased variability in patients' goals. A successful cosmetic surgeon will cultivate an understanding of aesthetic ideals in different ethnic groups, nurture discussions with patients to determine their aesthetic goals, devise a surgical plan for each patient, and develop and refine the necessary surgical skills to perform the procedure.

Facial plastic surgeons must understand nasal aesthetics in the context of race, ethnicity, and culture. The lack of aesthetic norms and ideal standards in non-Caucasian patients and the variation in nasal anatomy and morphology among races can create a challenge in approaching ethnic rhinoplasty. Preoperative assessment of nasal and facial features that contribute to a nose that is unpleasing for a non-Caucasian patient cannot be based on neoclassical canons. This article describes the concepts of facial aesthetics important to approaching ethnic rhinoplasty. Understanding these features will allow the surgeon to achieve nasal symmetry and improved definition without effacing ethnicity.

The motivations to pursue ethnically sensitive rhinoplasty and associated expectations are nuanced and influenced by the culture and institutional forces in a community. This article seeks to elucidate those nuances and the impact on self-image of patients seeking this procedure.

The nasal anatomy of Caucasian people includes thin skin, limited soft tissue volume, a high dorsum, strong cartilaginous framework, and narrow elliptical nasal inlets. A smooth dorsal contour, a well-defined tip, a naturally soft-feeling tip, and a functionally patent nasal valve constitute key objectives for Caucasian rhinoplasty. The author's focus on minimal-impact surgery has resulted in multiple novel techniques, embedded in a coherent algorithmic concept termed the S.O.F.T. (surgery and ongoing care free of trauma) concept. The foundation is the endonasal operation for the entire spectrum of primary and secondary deformities and maximal preservation of anatomic structures.

David A. Sherris

 Video content accompanies this article at http://www.oto.theclinics.com.

This article discusses common abnormalities found in the European or Caucasian nose. The treatments of the disorders via open structure rhinoplasty techniques are presented in a case-based manner. Multiple references are provided for further study of these techniques.

Hyung Gyun Na and Yong Ju Jang

Dorsal augmentation and tip surgery are essential procedures for East Asians seeking rhinoplasty, because they generally have thicker skin and poorly developed nasal dorsum and tip. For dorsal augmentation, many Asian surgeons prefer using alloplastic material, like silicone, Gore-Tex, and filler injection, for cost-effectiveness, easy handling, and short operation times. Compared with autologous implant materials, the use of synthetic implant is suggested to be associated with many complications, such as infection, extrusion, and deviation. However, even with the use of the autologous material, problems such as reabsorption after grafting, donor site complications can take place.

Roxana Cobo

Mestizo noses have mesorrhine nasal characteristics. They have a modest osteocartilaginous framework, nasal tips that tend to be bulbous with poor projection and rotation, and skins that tend to be thick and acne prone. A structural rhinoplasty approach is performed, focusing on anatomic findings. Conservative tissue excision with preservation or reinforcement of support structures of the nose is done. Structural grafting and suturing techniques are used to remodel cartilage and create better definition and support. The skin and soft tissue envelope is managed medically and surgically. The objective is to create balanced-looking noses that bring patients closer to their own aesthetic ideal.

Robert Deeb

Rhinoplasty in patients of Middle Eastern descent presents a unique challenge. There are a large number of variations of skin tone, skin thickness, and structural deformities, which require a high degree of thoughtfulness and planning. A thorough history and physical examination is the cornerstone to achieving a good result. An open and honest discussion is necessary to fully understand the patient's goals. The surgeon should clearly define which goals are achievable and which are not. Conservative techniques will help achieve a natural, balanced outcome and will allow for preservation of nasal function.

The US population increases yearly and by 2050, experts predict the US population will be greater than 430 million. As the population has grown, it has diversified and includes the largest percentage of multiethnic Americans to date. Accessibility and popularity of aesthetic surgery also have increased. Approaches to rhinoplasty have evolved from a concept of cultural and ethnic transformation to concepts of ethnic preservation, with the goal of preserving features while harmonizing the nose with the rest of the face. To achieve this goal thoughtful consultation and consideration of the patient's self-defined ethnicity is paramount.

Facial structure, nasal shape, and aesthetic nasal preferences vary broadly among patients of African descent who seek rhinoplasty. This variation reflects the broad diversity in this ethnic group and is highlighted by lapses in computer vision algorithms in accurately recognizing black faces. Across ethnicities, patients who seek rhinoplasty have similar goals: a reshaped nose that fits their facial features and enhances their facial beauty. Among patients of African descent, there is a particularly strong desire for maintaining nasal features that are ethnically sensitive and culturally congruent. This article discusses the nuances of managing the lower third of the African nose.

OTOLARYNGOLOGIC CLINICS
OF NORTH AMERICA

SERIES OF RELATED INTEREST

Facial Plastic Surgery Clinics
Available at: https://www.facialplastic.theclinics.com/

THE CLINICS ARE AVAILABLE ONLINE!
Access your subscription at:
www.theclinics.com

Foreword

Beauty is in the Eye of the Beholder and the Skill of the Surgeon

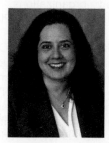

Sujana S. Chandrasekhar, MD, FACS, FAAOHNS
Consulting Editor

It wasn't very long ago that it seemed like every woman walking around the fancy shops in Manhattan looked eerily similar to every other one: they were all proudly sporting the same nose! In 1957, the Goldman tip was popularized. It is a vertical dome division endonasal approach that narrows the tip of the nose and causes a slightly upward projection. This results in a pert, adorable nose popularized by many American television stars in the 1960s and therefore coveted widely. The Diamond nose has that pert tip with a scooped-out bridge and was also widely popular in the 1960s and 1970s, again seemingly irrespective of the rest of the face. It is easy to see in hindsight that one nose does not fit all, and a tiny pert nose in the middle of a face with broader angles or other features may not result in the look that the patient actually wants. Drs Brissett, Ishii, and Boahene have compiled an impressive series of thoughtfully written articles examining ethnically sensitive approaches to rhinoplasty. This comprehensive issue of *Otolaryngologic Clinics of North America* features frank discussions of cultural ideals and detailed explanations of techniques.

The 1950s marked the beginning of otolaryngologists' entrance into the rhinoplasty arena. To understand why nasal tip work developed in the way that it did, we must go back to pre-Nazi Germany. Dr Jacques Joseph, an outstanding facial plastic and reconstructive surgeon, was a loyal German Jew.[1] His career began in Germany at the time of Emperor Wilhelm II, brought him the highest recognition as a doctor, and ended sadly under the National Socialists. As the Nazis gained power in Germany, medical officials became concerned that Dr Joseph was performing procedures either only for vanity's sake or, worse, in their estimation, in order to

Otolaryngol Clin N Am 53 (2020) ix–xi
https://doi.org/10.1016/j.otc.2020.01.002
0030-6665/20/© 2020 Published by Elsevier Inc.

camouflage Jews. His operating privileges were revoked throughout the city, even in Berlin's Jewish hospital, but his own clinic drew groups of apprentices from abroad who were permitted only to "observe" silently from the foot of the operating table. He died in 1934.

In post-war America, many of Dr Joseph's plastic surgery protégés flourished. His techniques changed the shape of the American nose for generations. However, like their professor, these physicians guarded their techniques closely. Dr Samuel Fomon[2] had also observed Dr Joseph's surgery. While plastic surgeons hid their work, he decided to teach otolaryngology residents and thus brought rhinoplasty into our field. He founded organizations, some of which went on to become the American Academy of Facial Plastic and Reconstructive Surgery.

Among Fomon's students at Mount Sinai Hospital in New York City was a young otolaryngologist named Irving Goldman. Goldman took techniques from Germany and the United States to develop his eponymous vertical dome division procedure.[3] A variation on this was the Dr Diamond nose, named for NYC doctor Howard Diamond. These were both omnipresent during the 1960s and 1970s. Look at any advertisement during those decades, and you will find ample examples of the Goldman and Diamond noses, in the center of various types of faces.

What began as techniques to change "ethnic" noses to make them conform to a "Caucasian ideal" of beauty has evolved over time. This is due to the appreciation that there is extraordinary beauty to be found not just in a narrow or pinched nose, but in a broad one as well, and that various skin and facial types need more critical and far-thinking approaches so that the surgeon and the patient are working toward the same goal.

Drs Brissett, Ishii, and Boahene, and the other authors, present us with a series of articles focusing on the personalization of rhinoplasty, with descriptions of various ethnic considerations in terms of facial skeleton and skin thickness and texture. The surgeon who has read these articles will find himself or herself better able to understand the patient's desires, counsel them more thoroughly, and end up with a satisfying cosmetic outcome of a beautiful and natural-appearing nose.[4] To quote John Kenneth Galbraith, "There is certainly no absolute standard of beauty. That precisely is what makes its pursuit so interesting."

Sujana S. Chandrasekhar, MD, FACS, FAAOHNS
Consulting Editor, Otolaryngologic Clinics of North America

Past President, American Academy of Otolaryngology-Head and Neck Surgery
Secretary-Treasurer, American Otological Society
Partner, ENT & Allergy Associates LLP
18 East 48th Street, 2nd Floor, New York, NY 10017, USA

Clinical Professor, Department of Otolaryngology-Head and Neck Surgery
Zucker School of Medicine at Hofstra-Northwell, Hempstead, NY, USA

Clinical Associate Professor, Department of Otolaryngology-Head and Neck Surgery
Icahn School of Medicine at Mount Sinai, New York, NY, USA

E-mail address:
ssc@nyotology.com

REFERENCES

1. Bhattacharya S. Jacques Joseph: father of modern aesthetic surgery. Indian J Plast Surg 2008;41(suppl):S3–8.
2. Bell JW. Pioneering physician: Samuel Fomon. Arch Otolaryngol 1971;94(5):387–8.
3. Goldman IB. The term "rhinoplasty". Eye Ear Nose Throat Mon 1955;34(4):258–9.
4. Glaser G. The nose: a profile of sex, beauty, and survival. New York: Washington Square Press; 2002.

Preface

Ethnically Sensitive Rhinoplasty

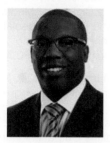   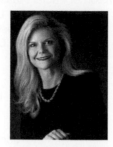   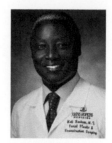

Anthony E. Brissett, MD, FACS   Lisa E. Ishii, MD, MHS   Kofi D.O. Boahene, MD, FACS
Editors

Over the past several decades, in the United States and around the world, we have witnessed a transformation in racial and cultural demographics and awareness. Within the United States, we have experienced population growth with significant increases seen in Hispanics, Asians, Indo-Asians, and patients of African descent. Greater social acceptance of cosmetic procedures and improved economics combined with this change in cultural demographics has resulted in an increase in individuals of diverse cultural backgrounds seeking cosmetic surgery.

Rhinoplasty is one of the most common procedures for patients of ethnic backgrounds seeking plastic surgery. This increase of ethnically diverse patients seeking rhinoplasty procedures is also accompanied by a shift in philosophy of the facial plastic surgeon performing rhinoplasty procedures on patients of ethnic descent. Over the past decades, we have witnessed a move away from western norms and ideas of beauty and a shift toward greater cultural awareness that is focused more on balance, harmony, symmetry, and the preservation of one's unique cultural facial features. With this in mind, we have also witnessed a transformation from rhinoplasty procedures that once resulted in cultural transformation and outcomes that embraced western ideas of beauty toward cultural or racial preservation and outcomes that promote the preservation of global concepts of beauty.

In this issue of *Otolaryngology Clinics of North America*, we explore the philosophies, strategies, and techniques of rhinoplasty with a focus on ethnic-sensitive rhinoplasty in pursuit of balance and harmony and cultural preservation. This issue is intended to allow the reader to review the techniques of experts that are aware of the subtleties of performing ethnic-sensitive rhinoplasty in the era of cultural and racial preservation.

As the editors of this issue, we would like to thank our authors, who have willing shared their expertise. To the reader, we thank you for taking the time to review the articles; we trust you will appreciate the expertise of our authors and be able to

Otolaryngol Clin N Am 53 (2020) xiii–xiv
https://doi.org/10.1016/j.otc.2020.01.001
0030-6665/20/© 2020 Published by Elsevier Inc.

oto.theclinics.com

incorporate the techniques shared in this issue for the benefit of your patients. Finally, we thank the Elsevier staff for their editing and assistance with this issue.

Anthony E. Brissett, MD, FACS
Department Otolaryngology/Head and Neck Surgery
Division of Facial Plastic and Reconstructive Surgery
Texas A&M University College of Medicine
Houston Methodist ENT Specialists
6550 Fannin Street, Suite 1703
Houston, TX 77030, USA

Lisa E. Ishii, MD, MHS
Department of Otolaryngology
Head & Neck Surgery
The Johns Hopkins University School of Medicine
Johns Hopkins Outpatient Center
601 North Caroline Street
Baltimore, MD 21287, USA

Kofi D.O. Boahene, MD, FACS
Otolaryngology Head and Neck Surgery
Division of Facial Plastic and Reconstructive Surgery
Department of Otolaryngology Head and Neck Surgery
The Johns Hopkins University School of Medicine
Johns Hopkins Outpatient Center
601 N. Caroline St, 6th Floor
Baltimore, MD 21287, USA

E-mail addresses:
aebrissett@houstonmethodist.org (A.E. Brissett)
learnes2@jhmi.ed (L.E. Ishii)
dboahen1@jhmi.edu (K.D.O. Boahene)

The Changing Face of Beauty
A Global Assessment of Facial Beauty

Katherine Elizabeth Hicks, MD[a],*, James Regan Thomas, MD[b]

KEYWORDS

- Global • Evolution • Facial beauty

KEY POINTS

- Despite the pervasive social, political, and economic effects of beauty, defining it is a struggle.
- Although generally there are some common tenets of facial beauty, it is important to recognize that there is significant variability in ideal facial features and proportions across different ethnic groups.
- It is extremely important that the surgeon be intimately familiar with each patient's individual concerns and goals and tailor the surgical plan accordingly rather than adopting a one-size-fits-all approach.

INTRODUCTION

Whether right or wrong, a great deal of importance is placed on beauty. When one sees another person, one assesses his or her appearance and often subconsciously judges his or her level of attractiveness. Over the years, people considered beautiful or handsome often enjoy certain advantages both socially and professionally. There are social, cultural, and economic influences inherent in the possession and endeavor of beauty.

Beauty has long been associated with positive attributes, while ugliness has been linked with negative characteristics. Studies have shown that attractive people are consistently rated as nicer, smarter, and healthier than their less attractive counterparts, and these findings have been consistent across different ages, sexual orientations, and ethnicities.[1–4] As far back as the seventh and eighth centuries BC, Saphho and Plato essentially proclaimed beauty to be synonymous with good and truth.[5] Today, Disney princes and princesses all typify common perceptions of beauty in culture. Conversely, villains are often portrayed as unattractive or somehow deformed,

[a] Department of Otolaryngology–Head & Neck Surgery, Northwestern University, 676 North Saint Clair Street, Suite 1325, Chicago, IL 60611, USA; [b] Facial Plastic and Reconstructive Surgery, Department of Otolaryngology–Head and Neck Surgery, Northwestern School of Medicine, 676 North Saint Clair Street, Suite 1325, Chicago, IL 60611, USA
* Corresponding author.
E-mail address: kehicks@ucdavis.edu

Otolaryngol Clin N Am 53 (2020) 185–194
https://doi.org/10.1016/j.otc.2019.12.005
0030-6665/20/© 2019 Elsevier Inc. All rights reserved.

oto.theclinics.com

perpetuating the association between ugly and evil. Despite myriad examples of beautiful people indulging in horrible activities or committing terrible crimes, one's first snap judgment of people with aesthetically pleasing faces is positive in most cases.

Despite the pervasive social, political, and economic effects of beauty, people often struggle to define it. People intuitively have a sense for what is beautiful, but its inherent subjectivity renders it difficult to define. The face signifies the consummate representation of a person, serving as each person's unique identifier. One remembers others primarily by their faces over any other physical attribute. Equally important, facial expressions are the primary medium through which voluntary and involuntary emotional expressions are conveyed.[6] The eyes and mouth are the most expressive elements of the face and are chiefly responsible for conveying a person's general mood.

It is generally accepted that the notion of facial beauty is complex. In 1 sense, it may be thought of as a purely subjective determination. Similar to renowned paintings in the artistic world, one may know a particular painting is beautiful but be unable to define precisely why it is beautiful. However, this is probably an overly simplistic approach to describing beauty.

On the other end of the spectrum, experts have long sought to delineate measurements, ratios, and characteristics that traverse cultural boundaries and universally represent beauty. The pursuit of a more objective definition of beauty has occupied physicians and other experts for centuries. In reality, the perception of beauty is largely subjective; however, there are objective aspects of facial analysis that, taken together, render a face more likely to be beautiful. As with many things in nature, there exists a combination of art and science; the concept of beauty is no different.

The population of the United States becomes more diverse by the day, and there are increasing numbers of interracial couples.[7] Thus, traditional stereotypes of beauty in various ethnic groups become less and less applicable as diversity increases. Often, new and uniquely beautiful facial features and proportions emerge as different ethnicities converge. With the increased diversity in facial appearance comes increased variability in patients' goals. One patient may wish to erase or minimize certain features, while another patient with the same features may wish to preserve or enhance them. It is extremely important that the surgeon be intimately familiar with each patient's individual concerns and goals and tailor the surgical plan accordingly rather than adopting a one-size-fits-all approach.

Despite the increasing heterogeneity of the population, there are a few key features that underlie most traditionally beautiful faces. These include: symmetry, averageness, youth, and sexual dimorphism. Through these factors, one can begin to assess beauty in a slightly more scientific and objective manner.

SYMMETRY AND BALANCE

Many people have investigated the role that symmetry plays in perception of facial beauty and found that, for both men and women, symmetric faces are rated as more attractive than faces with inherent asymmetries. It has been suggested that facial symmetry and attractiveness are directly correlated, but averageness of the symmetric faces may be a confounding factor in this finding.[8] Facial symmetry seems to confer an advantage in sexual competition,[9–12] as it has been purported to reflect a person's genetic and phenotypic condition.[13]

In keeping with the concept of symmetry and balance, the golden ratio, phi (approximately 1:1.618), is pervasive in nature and was believed by ancient Greeks to represent perfect harmony.[14,15] It is commonly found across ancient Egyptian art and architecture, and the ratio of consecutive numbers in the Fibonacci sequence converge to approximate phi. This ratio can be identified in many aspects of nature, from the proportion of arcs in a spiral-shaped seashell to the ratio of condylar to corpus axis growth in mandibles.[16,17]

In ancient Greece, the golden ratio was thought to apply to facial beauty also.[14] More recently, researchers have found that certain spatial ratios do tend to result in a more beautiful face, but these ratios are not consistently equivalent to the golden ratio.[18] The group presented series of faces in which all features, eyes, nose, and mouth, were identical, but horizontal and vertical distances between the features and facial length and width ratios were varied. A group of observers rated the attractiveness of each iteration in each series. Over the course of their simulations, they determined that attractiveness is optimized when the vertical distance between the eyes and the mouth is approximately 36% of facial length, and the horizontal distance between the eyes is approximately 46% of facial length.[18] The female face is thought to correspond with phi ratios better than the male face,[19] but even so, a female face whose length-to-width proportions are less than the golden ratio is considered more attractive than one whose proportions approximate phi.[20]

The pursuit to define ideal ratios is ongoing, and it is possible that there is no perfect objective measurement to define facial harmony. This is particularly true in light of the fact that, as people's ethnicities become more diverse and complex over time, the proportions that appear beautiful now may evolve.

AVERAGENESS

Although at first glance the relationship appears paradoxic, there are data to suggest that a face's beauty increases in parallel with its degree of averageness. Some believe averageness to be the defining characteristic of facial attractiveness in women.[8] To test this concept, one research group created a composite face from several individual faces and found that observers preferred the composite face to any of the individual faces.[1] Interestingly, utilization of increasing numbers of faces to generate a composite image correlated to increased attractiveness of the final image.[1] Another group performed similar studies, finding the same trend toward affinity for averageness for both the Caucasian female face and the Caucasian male face. The same group then performed composite imaging of Japanese faces and showed the images to Caucasian subjects and Japanese subjects; in both cases, the subjects tended to be more attracted to the average composite photo than any individual photo.[21]

This attraction to averageness again relates to Darwinian theories of evolution, which outline evolutionary bias against people at extremes of the population. Extrapolating from this, it can be inferred that those people closest to average represent genetic heterozygosity and a high probability of successfully passing their genes on.[22,23] Thus, it makes sense that averageness equates with beauty and that this principle is cross-cultural.

YOUTHFULNESS

If one stops to think about what features appear beautiful, one of the first features that comes to mind is often large eyes. Another feature commonly associated with beauty is a relatively small nose. One study digitally increased the size of women's eyes, and the modified images were consistently judged as more attractive than the original picture with smaller eyes.[2] Other studies demonstrated the same pattern of preference for youthful features across multiple different ethnic populations.[2–4]

Youthful features such as large eyes and small noses are characteristic of babies and young children; in general, neonatal features have been found to be suggestive of exuberance, amicability, and open-mindedness.[8] Thus, people likely subconsciously associate youthful features with these positive attributes.

During the aging process, volume is lost in the cheeks, and jowling occurs along the jawline. The brow descends, giving the eyes a hooded appearance and making them appear smaller. Taken together, these changes result in a sad or tired appearance.[24] The mind subconsciously interprets these changes as aging and, therefore, decreased fertility, decreasing overall attractiveness.

SEXUAL DIMORPHISM

Defined as the phenotypic differences between males and females, sexual dimorphism is another key feature that transcends different cultures to affect beauty universally. A high ratio of estrogen to testosterone is primarily responsible for the key differences between the male and female face and body. As women mature through adolescence, fat is deposited in the upper cheek, lips, breasts, and hips. The face elongates to a greater degree than it widens, creating a longer, narrower face. Taken together, these changes produce aesthetically-pleasing features: prominent eyes, high cheekbones, proportional nose, full lips, and relatively small chin. These characteristics are generally synonymous with femininity and increased fertility and result in an appearance that is, more desirable to the opposite sex.[2,8,22,25,26]

Similarly, high testosterone levels in men result in characteristically masculine features. These are often opposite in nature to attractive feminine features and include: thick hair, heavy brows, thin lips, and squared jawline with a strong chin. In general, women are attracted to these features, particularly those who are in their reproductive years.[26] Interestingly, as women age and are no longer seeking to reproduce, they seem to be attracted to slightly more feminized male face, which has been suggested to be a surrogate measure for their likelihood to remain invested in their relationships and in nurturing their families.[19,27]

BEAUTY ACROSS DIFFERENT CULTURES

Although there are the aforementioned common tenets of facial beauty, it is important to recognize that there is significant variability in ideal facial features and proportions across different ethnic groups. A recent systematic review aimed to evaluate the degree of variability in facial dimensions across many ethnic groups.[28] After application of exclusion criteria, the group analyzed 7 articles, comprising 2359 men and women from 27 different ethnic groups. The patients' ages ranged from 18 to 35 year old, and they had no history of craniofacial malformations, previous facial trauma, or previous facial surgery. These results reported the 11 linear facial measurements[29-31] traditionally included in the neoclassical canons described by Leonardo da Vinci and other European Renaissance artists (1452–1519 AD). The results of their analysis indicated that the greatest variation among ethnic groups was seen in forehead height, quantified as the distance between the trichion and the nasion. Although the width of the malar region (interzygion distance) and the distance between the lateral canthi (interexocanthion distance) were the least variable, the intercanthal distance (interendocanthion distance) was variable.

Another study sought to compile normative data regarding facial measurements in various ethnic groups around the world.[32] Data were collected by scientists experienced in anthropometric measurements. The collected data were compared with the established norms of North American Caucasians. The group identified 1470 healthy subjects (750 men, 720 women), aged 18 to 30 years, from Europe (n = 780), the Middle East (n = 180), Asia (n = 300), and Africa (n = 210). Fourteen anthropometric measurements were taken, including the neoclassical canons described by da Vinci and others. The group found that the greatest differences among different ethnic groups were seen in the measurements of the orbital region. Nasal height and width exhibited significant variation. Asian and African-American groups were found to have very to extremely significantly wide noses when compared with Caucasians. In the Middle Eastern patients, the nasal width was similar to Caucasians, but the height was significantly greater.

Although there is much work to be done in describing the facial features of various ethnic groups, there is now increased awareness of variability among different ethnic groups and the importance of preserving and enhancing each group's unique features. This is pertinent in all areas of cosmetic surgery, as the surgical goals and techniques may be vastly different for patients of different ethnicities. In no area of cosmetic facial surgery is this more apparent than in ethnic rhinoplasty, and it is exceedingly important that a facial plastic surgeon be knowledgeable regarding the different aesthetic goals and challenges in these patients.

ETHNIC RHINOPLASTY
Principles and Popularity

For many years, the concept of what constitutes the ideal nose was based on the overall appearance, contours, and angles of the aesthetically pleasing Caucasian nose. In the idealized Caucasian nose, the dorsum is straight, smooth, and appropriately projected. The radix is 3 or 4 mm deep and located at the level of the upper lid crease. The overall length of the nose takes up approximately one-third of the vertical distance of the face. The nasal tip is proportional, symmetric, and well-defined, and the nasal base is optimally located between the medial canthi or perhaps just slightly wider. From a structural standpoint, the upper and lower lateral cartilages are relatively strong, and the nasal bones are typically moderate in length, although there is some variation.

In the United States, the last few decades have seen a marked increase in the number of non-Caucasian patients undergoing cosmetic surgery procedures. From 2008 to 2018, the number of African-American, Hispanic, and Asian patients undergoing cosmetic procedures increased 76%, 52%, and 39%, respectively.[33,34] As these figures continue to rise, it becomes increasingly important that surgeons maintain an appreciation for and technical knowledge of the different aesthetic goals and functional considerations when performing cosmetic surgery in these patients.

When cosmetic surgery started gaining in popularity among people of various ethnicities, early attempts at rhinoplasty in these groups were often performed with the aforementioned ideals based on the Caucasian nose. This strategy led to both aesthetic and functional problems in non-Caucasian rhinoplasty. Now, it is widely recognized that people of different ethnicities have different aesthetic ideals from many Caucasian patients. Additionally, there are often structural differences in the underlying nasal framework that surgeons must take into consideration from a functional standpoint. **Table 1** summarizes some of the more consistent and prominent characteristics of nasal anatomy in each ethnic group described herein. However, it should be emphasized that, across all ethnicities, the principle goals of rhinoplasty remain the same: improving nasal and facial harmony and symmetry, improving or maintaining function, preserving unique, defining characteristics of each ethnicity to the extent desired by the patient, and maintaining a natural appearance.

Table 1
Characteristic features of nasal anatomy in different ethnic groups

	Skin and Soft Tissue Envelope	Bony Framework	Cartilaginous Framework	Nasal Dorsum	Nasal Tip, Alae, and Base
African-American	Moderately to very thick skin	Short[a], wide nasal bones Less prominent premaxilla and anterior nasal spine	Weak Moderately poor tip support	Wide Low dorsum	Acute nasolabial angle Short columella Wide, poorly defined tip Broad nasal base Thick nasal alae, often with excess flare
Hispanic	Moderate-to-thick skin	Short, slightly wide nasal bones	Weak, thin Poor tip support	Low dorsum	Tip underprojected Short columella Wide, poorly defined tip Broad nasal base Thick nasal alae, often with excess flare Nostrils horizontally oriented
Asian	Moderate-to-thick skin Higher collagen density	Variable length of nasal bones	Moderately poor tip support	Shallow radix Low dorsum	Tip underprojected Wide nasal tip Columellar retraction
Middle Eastern	Thick, sebaceous skin	Wide nasal bones	Moderate tip support	Long dorsum Dorsal hump	Acute nasolabial angle Relative deficiency in tip projection Bulbous, poorly defined tip Prominent infratip lobule

[a] Denotes functional implications.

Patient Evaluation

When a patient presents for rhinoplasty consultation, it is equally important to closely examine and critically analyze the patient's nose and have a detailed discussion regarding the patient's aesthetic and functional goals. When examining the patient, it is important to keep aesthetic and structural considerations in mind. From an aesthetic standpoint, the surgeon should evaluate the nose from multiple viewpoints and make note of particular features on each view. **Table 2** summarizes the most important components to evaluate on each of the principle nasal views. When trying to delineate a patient's aesthetic goals, it may be helpful to ask what his or her family members' noses look like and which features he or she would like to change or maintain. The surgeon should also consider offering adjunct procedures that may further enhance the patient's appearance, such as chin augmentation in patients with microgenia. Additionally, high-quality photography and regular use of image morphing software are critical components to optimize communication between surgeon and patient during consultation. Regular use of morphed images provides the patient with realistic images of the intended final appearance and allows the surgeon to ensure that he or she fully understands the patient's goals.

During cosmetic rhinoplasty, it is tempting to focus predominantly on the aesthetic outcome, but a good functional result is equally important. Careful evaluation of the patient's septum should reveal the presence of deviation, spurs, and perforations, if present. It will also provide important information regarding the quantity and strength of available cartilage, which may signal the need to plan on using a secondary source of cartilage for grafting purposes, such as auricular or rib cartilage. The integrity and strength of the upper and lower lateral cartilages should be assessed, as weak cartilages are partially responsible for compromised internal and external nasal valve function. This is particularly important to bear in mind during preparation for ethnic rhinoplasty. The cartilage in these patients tends to be weaker than in Caucasians,

Table 2
Essential examination components on each principle view of the nose

View	Important Features and Measurements
Frontal	Overall length of nose Overall symmetry Presence of irregularity or deformity Brow-tip aesthetic line Width of nasal dorsum Width and contour of nasal tip Width of nasal base Degree of alar flaring, if present
Profile	Overall length of nose Location and depth of radix Contour and projection of dorsum Tip rotation, projection, and contour Alar-lobule ratio Alar-columellar relationship Chin size and projection
Base	Symmetry of tip and nostrils Degree of caudal deviation, if present Tip configuration and triangularity Columellar-lobule ratio

and, in many ethnic groups, many intended rhinoplasty maneuvers are reductive in nature. In these patients, a surgeon must recognize that overly aggressive reductive maneuvers in the absence of appropriate structural modification will almost certainly lead to nasal valve collapse and difficulty breathing postoperatively.

Nasal Anatomy and Aesthetics in Ethnic Rhinoplasty

Table 1 summarizes the typical characteristics of the African-American, Hispanic, Asian, and Middle Eastern nose. Each presents its own unique challenges, but there are a few key aspects that are common to these ethnic groups. The first of these commonalities is the tendency toward thicker, often more sebaceous skin. This is often a clinically limiting factor in the pursuit of tip reduction and refinement. Additionally, the thickness and bulk of skin and soft tissue may compromise nasal function in the setting of weaker cartilages in the nasal tip. In many cases, some degree of debulking is necessary to achieve desired refinement in the tip. However, it is important to be conservative and avoid disrupting the subdermal plexus, which may lead to devascularization or even necrosis of the skin. One advantage of thicker skin is that it does tend to camouflage some minor irregularities that might otherwise be evident after edema has resolved.

Additionally, the upper and lower lateral cartilages tend to be thinner and weaker than those encountered in Caucasian rhinoplasty. This is particularly important to bear in mind, because the desired aesthetic result in ethnic rhinoplasty often requires reductive maneuvers. The surgeon must plan carefully, implementing conservative reduction, reinforcing maneuvers, or a combination thereof.

In these groups, the bony dorsum is often wide. To achieve a narrower profile may require aggressive osteotomies or, in some cases, a dorsal onlay graft to give the illusion of a narrower dorsum on frontal view. Similarly, the nasal tip is commonly wide and often poorly defined. Refinement of the tip without compromise of tip support or nasal valve integrity requires thoughtful surgical planning.

It is important to emphasize that, although these groups frequently share common features and characteristics, significant variation exists within and among these different groups. A successful rhinoplasty surgeon will carefully evaluate each individual patient's unique features and tailor the surgical plan accordingly.

SUMMARY

The United States is becoming more and more diverse by the day, and cosmetic surgery is gaining in popularity across all ethnic groups. A successful cosmetic surgeon will: cultivate a thorough understanding of aesthetic ideals in different ethnic groups, nurture open and honest discussions with each patient to determine his or her unique aesthetic goals, devise a thoughtful, comprehensive surgical plan for each patient, and develop and refine the necessary surgical skills to successfully perform the procedure.

DISCLOSURE

The authors have nothing to disclose.

REFERENCES

1. Langlois J, Roggman L. Attractive faces are only average. Psychol Sci 1990;1: 115–21.

2. Cunningham M, Roberts A, Barbee A, et al. "Their ideas of beauty are, on the whole, the same as ours": consistency and variability in the crosscultural perception of female attractiveness. J Pers Soc Psychol 1995;68:261–79.
3. Jones D, Hill K. Criteria of facial attractiveness in five populations. Hum Nat 1993; 4:271–96.
4. Jones D, Brace CL, Jankowiak W, et al. Sexual selection, physical attractiveness, and facial neoteny: cross-cultural evidence and implications. Curr Anthropol 1995;36(5):723–48.
5. Hoerber R. Plato's greater hippias. Phronesis 1969;9(2):143–55.
6. Synnott A. The beauty mystique. Facial Plast Surg 2006;22(3):163–74.
7. Kridel R. Ethnicity in facial plastic surgery. Facial Plast Surg 2010;26:61–2.
8. Baudouin J, Tiberghien G. Symmetry, averageness, and feature size in the facial attractiveness of women. Acta Psychol 2004;117:313–32.
9. Gangestad S, Thornhill R, Yeo R. Facial attractiveness, developmental stability, and fluctuating asymmetry. Ethol Sociobiol 1994;15:73–85.
10. Grammer K, Thornhill R. Human facial attractiveness and sexual selection: the role of averageness and symmetry. J Comp Psychol 1994;108:233–42.
11. Thornhill R, Gangestad S. Human facial beauty: averageness, symmetry, and parasite resistance. Hum Nat 1993;4:237–69.
12. Mealey L, Bridgstock R, Townsend G. Symmetry and perceived facial attractiveness: a monozygomatic co-twin comparison. J Pers Soc Psychol 1999;76: 157–65.
13. Wayneforth D. Fluctuating asymmetry and human male life-history traits in rural Belize. Proc Biol Sci 1998;265:1497–501.
14. Atalay B. Math and the Mona Lisa: the art and science of Leonardo Da Vinci. New York: Harper Collins Publishers; 2006.
15. Prokopakis E, Vlastos I, Picavet V, et al. The golden ratio in facial symmetry. Rhinology 2013;51(1):18–21.
16. Thompson D. On growth and form. New York: Dover; 1992.
17. Cook T. The curves of life. New York: Dover; 1978.
18. Pallett P, Link S, Lee K. New "golden" ratios for facial beauty. Vis Res 2010;50: 149–54.
19. Bashour M. An objective system for measuring facial attractiveness. Plast Reconstr Surg 2006;118(3):757–74.
20. Schmid K, Marx D, Samal A. Computation of a face attractiveness index based on neoclassical canons, symmetry, and golden ratios. Pattern Recogn 2008;41: 2710–7.
21. Perrett D, May K, Yoshikawa S. Facial shape and judgments of female attractiveness. Nature 1994;368:239–42.
22. Thornhill R, Gangestad S. Facial attractiveness. Trends Cogn Sci 1999;3:452–60.
23. Penton-Voak I, Perrett D. Consistency and individual differences in facial attractiveness judgments: an evolutionary perspective. Soc Res (New York) 2000;67: 219–44.
24. Knoll B, Attkiss K, Persing J. The influence of forehead, brow, and periorbital aesthetics on perceived expression in the youthful face. Plast Reconstr Surg 2008; 121:1793.
25. Cunningham M. Measuring the physical in physical attractiveness: quasi-experiments on the sociobiology of female facial beauty. J Pers Soc Psychol 1986;50:925–35.
26. Keating C. Gender and the physiognomy of dominance and attractiveness. Soc Psychol Q 1985;48:61.

27. Weeks D, Thomas J. Beauty in a multicultural world. Facial Plast Surg Clin North Am 2014;22:337–41.
28. Fang F, Clapham P, Chung K. A systematic review of interethnic variability in facial dimensions. Plast Reconstr Surg 2011;127(2):874–81.
29. Farkas L, Forrest C, Litsas L. Revision of neoclassical facial canons in young adult Afro-Americans. Aesthetic Plast Surg 2000;24:179–84.
30. Farkas L, Hreczko T, Kolar J, et al. Vertical and horizontal proportions of the face in young adult North American Caucasians: revision of neoclassical canons. Plast Reconstr Surg 1985;75:328–38.
31. Vegter F, Hage J. Clinical anthropometry and canons of the face in historical perspective. Plast Reconstr Surg 2000;106:1090–6.
32. Farkas L, Katic M, Forrest C. International anthropometric study of facial morphology in various ethnic groups/races. J Craniofac Surg 2005;16(4):615–46.
33. Plastic surgery statistics report. 2008. Available at: https://www.plasticsurgery.org/documents/News/Statistics/2008/plastic-surgery-statistics-full-report-2008.pdf. Accessed August 31, 2019.
34. Plastic surgery statistics report. 2018. Available at: https://www.plasticsurgery.org/news/plastic-surgery-statistics. Accessed August 31, 2019

Concepts of Facial Aesthetics When Considering Ethnic Rhinoplasty

Priyesh N. Patel, MD, Sam P. Most, MD*

KEYWORDS

- Ethnic rhinoplasty • African American rhinoplasty • East Asian rhinoplasty
- Middle Eastern rhinoplasty • Hispanic rhinoplasty • Facial aesthetics

KEY POINTS

- The lack of clear aesthetic norms and ideal standards in non-Caucasian patients and the variation in nasal morphology among races makes ethnic rhinoplasty challenging.
- Assessment of nasal and facial features that contribute to a nose that is unpleasing for a non-Caucasian patient cannot be based on neoclassical canons.
- Understanding the nasal features common to different racial groups, along with a patient's aesthetic goals, allows for optimal rhinoplasty results without effacing ethnicity.

INTRODUCTION

The racial and ethnic diversity of the United States has changed considerably over the course of the past century and is expected to continue to evolve over the next several decades. The United States population is expected to grow by 24.8% between 2016 and 2060, and while the Caucasian majority is expected to grow by 10.5%, the African American, Asian, and Hispanic populations are expected to grow by 40.6%, 100.8%, and 93.2% respectively.[1] This population change and growing global appeal for aesthetic facial plastic surgery will significantly impact the profile of patients seeking cosmetic surgery. Surveys from the American Academy of Facial Plastic and Reconstructive Surgery have demonstrated increased requests for cosmetic facial surgery among racial minority groups.[2] By the year 2030, 32% of all aesthetic procedures are expected to be performed on patients from a race other than Caucasian.[3] Of these procedures, rhinoplasty is considered one of the most popular sought out by non-Caucasian ethnic groups. With the increasing diversity in patients seeking facial rejuvenation procedures, facial plastic surgeons will need to develop a clear understanding of

Division of Facial Plastic and Reconstructive Surgery, Stanford University School of Medicine, 801 Welch Road, Stanford, CA 94304, USA
* Corresponding author.
E-mail address: smost@stanford.edu

Otolaryngol Clin N Am 53 (2020) 195–208
https://doi.org/10.1016/j.otc.2019.12.001
oto.theclinics.com

facial aesthetics in the context of race, ethnicity, and culture. This insight is imperative to surgical planning and ultimately patient satisfaction in rhinoplasty.

DEFINING THE GOALS OF ETHNIC RHINOPLASTY

Throughout literature, the term ethnic rhinoplasty is commonly used to refer to rhinoplasty in the non-Caucasian population. This includes patients of African, East Asian (eg, Korean, Chinese, Japanese, and Filipino), Middle Eastern (eg, Persian/Iranian, and Arab), and Hispanic (eg, Castilian or Mexican American) descent. As such, the term ethnic rhinoplasty is not a single entity, but rather a generic term with many inherent complexities.[4] These complexities can present a challenge for facial plastic surgeons and arise from a multitude of factors, including: unclear understanding of race, culture, and ethnicity as they apply to a patient's aesthetic goal; lack of clear aesthetic norms and ideal standards in non-Caucasian patients; and variation in nasal anatomy and morphology among and within races.

Race is an objective term that allows grouping based on biologic and physical similarities among a population of people. This is distinct from ethnicity, which is a subjective term that refers to a patient's personal sense of connection to a group and may be based on similarities in cultural beliefs and practices.[5] Therefore, patients of the same race may identify with different ethnic groups, and generalizations concerning race are not always in harmony with the subjective views held by members of the group.[2] It is therefore imperative that a surgeon explore the interplay between race and ethnicity of a patient, in addition to his or her personal concept of beauty, to determine the ultimate aesthetic goals of a patient.

It is the responsibility of an aesthetic rhinoplasty surgeon to help guide a patient, regardless of race, to determine what nasal and facial features contribute to a nose that is undesirable for the patient. The standard of beauty for the Caucasian face is based on neoclassical canons detailing ideal proportions, angles, and relationships between facial landmarks (**Fig. 1**).[6–12] For example, the ideal nasolabial angle among Caucasian women is 95° to 110°, and the alar base width is equivalent to the intercanthal distance. Although these rules were developed by artists, they have been widely taught and implemented by aesthetic surgeons to guide refinement of the Caucasian nose. Although several authors have used anthropometric or photogrammetric measurements to determine average facial measurements among subsets of non-Caucasian populations, no well-established ideal standard has been implemented for African, Asian, Hispanic, or Middle Eastern noses.[13–16] Moreover, classic anthropometric measurements, even in Caucasian patients, are based on average data acquired from general populations and not necessarily those considered attractive.[17] The aesthetic surgeon is then challenged to counsel patients without a universal standard or race-specific ideal of beauty to guide decision making.

A potential mistake is to apply the ideal facial proportions and relationships in the Caucasian face to the ethnic rhinoplasty. This so-called racial transformation of the nose is a historic concept and not recommended by the senior author and other leading rhinoplasty surgeons. However, an important consideration is that although most patients will wish to maintain a varying degree of ethnic expression, others will desire a nose more in line with neoclassical canons based on personal concepts of beauty that are influenced by the patient's social circle.[18] The aesthetic surgeon must also understand that patients in the United States may be comparing their noses with nonsimilar races, and this can lead to unrealistic desires. Establishing clear goals on behalf of the patient is essential to preventing postoperative dissatisfaction and limiting the need for revision ethnic restoration rhinoplasty.[19]

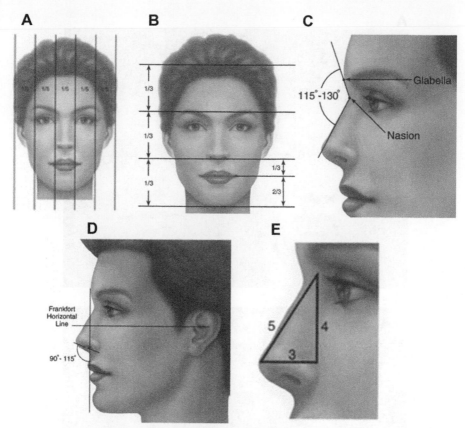

Fig. 1. Ideal nasal and facial features based on neoclassical canons. (*A*) The face is divided into facial fifths by vertical lines. (*B*) The face is divided into vertical thirds by horizontal lines. The intercanthal distance is equal to the width of the alar base. (*C*) The nasofrontal angle is typically 115° to 130°. (*D*) The nasolabial angle should be 90° to 95° in men and 95° to 115° in women. (*E*) Nasal projection and length illustrated as a 3–4–5 triangle. (*From*: Papel, I., et al. Facial Plastic and Reconstructive Surgery. Thieme: New York. 2016. p. 340, 373-4, 378.)

The goal of ethnic rhinoplasty, just like rhinoplasty in Caucasian patients, is to improve objective beauty of a person's face as determined by the harmony of proportions and symmetry without effacing ethnicity. Although the neoclassical canons are rarely even found in beautiful Caucasian faces, significant disproportions and disharmonies are more commonly found in faces considered less attractive.[20] Therefore, assessment of the nose in relation to other facial landmarks in the absence of ideal standards is important. Notably, although reduction rhinoplasty is commonly performed in the Western population, ensuring facial balance in ethnic populations may require augmentation in one area, which could decrease the amount of overall reduction necessary in another area (**Fig. 2**).[21] Ultimately, it is imperative that the surgeon work to improve definition, while ensuring preservation of ethnic features and that an individual's perception of beauty is achieved. This fundamentally requires an understanding of certain anatomic and morphologic features that are common to different racial groups. This is not without a caveat.

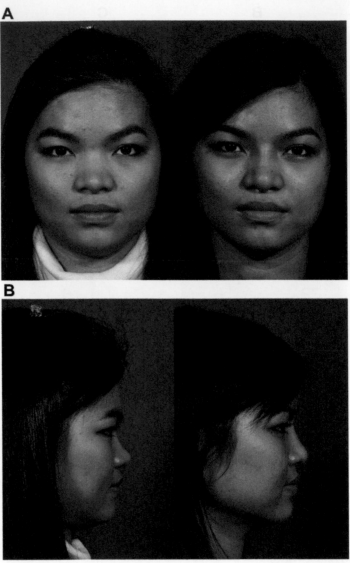

Fig. 2. An example of preoperative (*left*) and postoperative (*right*) augmentation rhinoplasty as seen on frontal (*A*) and lateral (*B*) views.

In the era of globalization, changes in migration patterns, and interracial marriages, attempts to define racial facial morphology will grow increasingly difficult. In response to this, Cobo suggests that noses can be anatomically divided into 3 generalized groups (mesorrhine, platyrrhine, and leptorrhine) and that most noses will have a mixture of these characteristics (**Fig. 3**).[5] The platyrrhine noses are common in patients of African descent and characterized by small nasal bones with a low radix and wide dorsum, flattened cartilaginous framework at the midvault, reduced tip support with decreased projection, acute nasolabial angles, and thick soft tissue envelope. The leptorrhine nose is typical in Caucasian patients and is on the opposite end of the anatomic spectrum relative to platyrrhine noses. The nasal bones are well developed with a high radix, and the

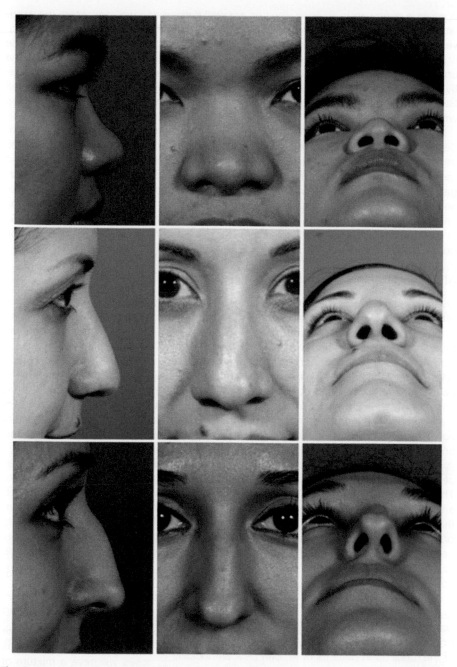

Fig. 3. Examples of the platyrrhine (*top row*), mesorrhine (*middle row*), and leptorrhine (*bottom row*) nasal morphology in lateral (*left column*), frontal (*middle column*), and basal (*right column*) views.

dorsum is narrower. In addition, the tips are well defined and well projected; the naso-labial angles have a slightly obtuse angle with adequate rotation, and the soft tissue envelope is thin with an underlying strong osseocartilaginous framework. The mesorrhine nose is common in Hispanic populations and has features in between the leptorrhine and platyrrhine nose. It is characterized by an osseocartilaginous framework that is relatively weaker than the Caucasian nose, but stronger than the platyrrhine noses. The soft tissue envelope is of intermediate thickness, and the tip lacks some degree of projection with acute nasolabial angles.

Although this strategy allows one to globally think of and categorize noses, an understanding of nasal and facial features within distinct racial groups will arm the aesthetic surgeon with the knowledge to transform noses in a patient-centered and sensitive manner. The problem of other race face perception, based on inherent surgeon bias, introduces the possibility that a surgeon who belongs to 1 race may be less sensitive to the distinguishing facial features of another ethic group.[21] The following sections are therefore meant to provide a summary of the nasal and facial aesthetic in the African, Hispanic, East Asian, and Middle Eastern population that should be considered during the ethnic rhinoplasty.

AFRICAN AMERICAN RHINOPLASTY

Over the last several decades, African American rhinoplasty has received critical attention as the disastrous and racially incongruent results of well-known African American celebrities have come to light. A survey of 196 African American patients found that that most patients do not want their nasal modifications to resemble Caucasian noses and that common complaints are that the nose is too broad or wide.[22] Although several authors have identified significant anatomic variability among the African American population based on origin, several anatomic features appear to be consistently seen among this group.[23,24] As such, 5 overarching goals in African American rhinoplasty have been previously summarized as follows: maintaining nasal-facial harmony and balance; ensuring a narrower, straight dorsum; enhancing tip projection and definition; maintaining slight alar flaring; and narrowing interalar distance.[25]

The nasal skin in African American patients, regardless of origin, is thick and sebaceous, and there is an abundance of fibrofatty tissue relative to the Caucasian nose. This is particularly notable at the nasal tip, which contributes to a loss in tip definition and bulbosity. The subcutaneous tissue typically measures between 2 to 4 mm in thickness.[25] The underlying cartilaginous framework may therefore not be easily palpable on preoperative assessment, and intraoperative structural refinement may be less visible postoperatively. In addition, as the skin has an inelastic nature, there can be a limit on the augmentation and tip projection that is feasible for a particular patient.[26]

Although the lower lateral cartilages in African Americans have previously been described as relatively short and weak, 2 studies have found that the integrity and size of the cartilage are similar to the Caucasian nose.[25,27] In addition, the distance from the caudal edge of the lower lateral cartilages to the alar rim is similar.[27] Nuances of the nasal tip in patients of African descent include

An obtuse intradomal distance which results in a broader, less defined, and less projected appearing tip

An acute lateral crural cartilage angle of inclination relative to the maxilla, which results in an underrotated appearance

A less prominent nasal spine and shorter columella, which contributes to decreased projection[24,27,28]

Despite the retruded maxillary spine, many African Americans have bimaxillary protrusion and relative microgenia. These features should be noted preoperatively, as chin implantation may be considered.[25] In reported comparisons of anthropometric measures, the nasolabial angles (degrees) in African American and Caucasian noses have been 86 to 91 versus 99 in women and 83.1 to 83.5 versus 98.9 to 99.8 in men, respectively.[13,29,30]

In a cadaveric study of skulls, the nasal bones in African patients have been found to be shorter and have an obtuse angle between each other, resulting in a flatter and broader appearance of the dorsum.[31] The mean width of the nasal root in African Americans is 25 to 27 mm compared with 15 to 16 mm in Caucasians.[29,30] The radix is deeper set, and although it is thought that the nasofrontal angle is more obtuse than the neoclassical teaching of 120°, there is a variation in comparative reports of nasofrontal angles (degrees) between African American and Caucasian patients (male: 126.9–135.6 vs 130–130.5; females: 131.9–133 vs 134, respectively).[13,29,30] The increased bony width is also translated into a broader cartilaginous midvault.

The pyriform aperture shape is variable in African Americans, but in general is more ovoid and with a shorter vertical height compared with Caucasians.[29,31] This contributes to a wider nasal base. It is important to note that despite the wider root and base of the nose, the relationship between the two has been found to be similar between attractive African American and Caucasian women (62% vs 60%).[29] Compared with the traditional teaching of a 1:1 relationship between intercanthal distance and nasal base width, Porter and colleagues[13,30] found a relationship of 1:1.25 and 1:3 in African American women and men. Therefore, an intracaruncular distance is perhaps more accurate in assessing the appropriate width of the African American nose. In addition, a more horizontal orientation of the lower lateral cartilages causes a portion of the alar typically to flare beyond the alar base attachment in African Americans by more than 2 mm, and as the aesthetic surgeon plans on nasal tip refinement or alar base reduction, attempts at maintaining some alar flare is imperative.[10,25] A wide range of nostril shapes have been described in African Americans, and the orientation is commonly more horizontal than is seen in Caucasians and may even take on an inverted shape such that the most lateral apex is oriented toward the tip rather the nasal base.[23] The columella to tip lobule relationship is therefore usually 1.4 to 1.5:1, which is shorter than the classic 2:1 ratio.[13,24,30]

MESTIZO/HISPANIC RHINOPLASTY

The terms Hispanic, Latinx, and Mestizo have been used interchangeably to describe patients from Spanish-speaking countries, and as such there is a wide variation of nasal morphology seen among this group. The nasal structure in mestizos has shared features with the European, African, and Indian noses.[32] As such, generalizations that can be made for the African American nose are more difficult to make for the Hispanic nose.

Ortiz-Monasterio, a pioneer in Hispanic rhinoplasty, identified 5 characteristics to be primary factors that differentiate mestizo noses from Caucasian noses.[33] First, similar to the African American nose, Hispanic noses have a thicker, more sebaceous, soft-tissue envelope. Second, these patients have a relatively small osseocartilaginous vault with wider but shorter nasal bones. Third, because of short medial crura and a weak caudal septum, the tip has less support and appears less projected and rotated. Fourth, the columella is typically hidden with a shorter membranous septum. Finally, Hispanic patients have a broader alar base with slight alar flaring. Additional features of the anthropologically termed mesorrhine nose have been used to describe the

Hispanic nose and differentiate it from that of Caucasians.[21,34,35] These include broader faces with prominent malar eminences, more horizontally oriented nostrils, a more acute nasolabial angle but similar nasofacial angle, higher base width to inter-canthal ratio, and greater midface protrusion but more recession of the lower face. A prevalence of dorsal humps is seen in the Hispanic population. However, these may be pseudohumps made apparent by the lack of tip protrusion or a lower radix position. Importantly, the prominence of the premaxilla can contribute to a more acute nasola-bial angle seen in Hispanic patients, and the tip may not actually be ptotic in relation-ship to the face.[21] As such, the nasolabial angle many not be an accurate method of assessing tip rotation in the Hispanic patient.

Attempts have been made to better describe the large variation in nasal architecture found among the Hispanic population. In an initial anthropometric analysis of Latinx noses compared with Caucasian and African American noses, Milgrim and col-leagues[14] identified 3 distinct Hispanic groups based on origin: Caribbean, Central American, and South American. The Caribbean population had noses resembling the anthropometric normative features of the African American, nose while the Central and South American noses had features more similar to Caucasians. Subsequently, Daniel proposed a different classification consisting of 3 nasal types: Castilian, Mexican American, and mestizo, and this was reinforced by Higuera and colleagues,[36] who similarly identified 3 archetypes of Hispanic noses.[37] Although these studies lack precise comparative anthropometric measurements, they provide a useful facial anal-ysis tool for the aesthetic surgeon.

As a summary of reported findings, patients in the first archetype or Castilian profile have a variable skin thickness that is thinner than the African American population. The radix is generally in a high to normal position with prominent nasal bones, and there is a high arched osseocartilaginous dorsum. Although the tip projection is similar to the Caucasian population, the tip width may appear slightly wide, and there is variability in the width of the base. Patients in the second archetype or Mexican American profile also have a variable skin thickness, but unlike the first group, have a lower radix posi-tion. Although the bony dorsum is not prominent, a decreased tip projection results in the illusion of a major dorsal hump. Noticing this is imperative, as a dorsal reduction may not be appropriate for this group of patients. The remainder of the nose shares features with the Caucasian nose. The third archetype or mestizo nose has features that more closely resemble the Caribbean population as described by Milgrim and col-leagues. The nasal skin is thicker with more abundant fibrofatty tissue. The alar base and the dorsum are wider than would be seen in Caucasian patients. The nasal tip is less projected and has a loss of definition, features similar to the African American population. These classification schemes reinforce an important element of rhino-plasty in the Hispanic patient; a large variability in structural morphology requires an individualized approach to nasal refinement.

EAST ASIAN RHINOPLASTY

The nasal profile in the East Asian population, consisting of those from China, Korea, Japan, and many parts of southeast Asia, has been broadly classified as mesorrhine.[16] It therefore follows that similar to Hispanic patients, the nasal skin is thicker than Caucasian patients. Mean thickness of the soft tissue envelope over the radix/nasal bones is 3.1 mm, and over the alar cartilage is 5.7 mm.[38] The alar lobule is particularly prominent in East Asian patients, with a dense underlying muscular and fatty layer without underlying cartilage. Although the nostril floor width is similar between East Asians and Caucasians, the interalar distance is greater (males: 39.5 mm vs

34.7 mm; females: 37.6 mm vs 31.4 mm, respectively).[16] This is attributed to the thick, flaring alar lobules. Notably, as is seen in attractive Caucasian faces, the intercanthal distance has been found to be similar to the interalar distance is attractive East Asian faces.[17] The junction of the cheek with the alar lobule is typically at or below the level of the columella insertion, resulting in a hidden collumela.[16] On base view, the orientation of the nostrils is typically more horizontal.

The ratio between nasal length and dorsal height is 2:0.61 in East Asians compared with 2:1 in Caucasians.[39] The radix is positioned lower, and the nasal dorsum is shorter and wider in East Asians, with a gentle curve rather than a distinct ridge as is seen in Caucasians.[16] These features result in a relatively underprojected and broader-appearing nose in the middle and upper portions. The tip is similarly broader and bulbous in appearance, in part because of the increased distance between the nasal domes and the thicker soft tissue envelope.[40] A shorter columellar segment of the medial crura results in a less projected nose. Nasal tip protrusion (subnasale to nasal tip) measures 16 to 17 mm in East Asians compared with 19 to 20 mm in Caucasians.[16] Although the alar cartilages in Asians are considered thin and weak in relation to the overlaying soft tissue, the average length of the lateral crus is similar to that seen in Caucasians (18 mm).[40]

The nasofrontal angle in East Asian patients is slightly greater than Caucasians (male: 137 vs 130°, female: 139 vs 134°).[16] Conflicting measures in regards to the nasolabial angle in Asians exist in the literature.[16,17,40–42] In a study using indirect laser scan measurements in East Asians, the nasolabial angle was measured to be obtuse (males: 99.9°, females: 97.7°) and more similar to direct anthropometric measures in Caucasians (males: 98.9°, females: 99.1°).[16] However, other studies, including direct anthropometric measures in Asian populations, have reported more acute nasolabial angles.[16,40,42] In a recent evaluation of attractive faces, the ideal nasolabial angle was found to be 109.5° in East Asians compared with 101.8° in Caucasians.[17] This represents a distinction from the classic messorhine nasal morphology.

Attempts have been made to create classification schemes within the Asian population to account for variability and help the surgeon determine what surgical interventions may be appropriate. Aung and colleagues[16] found that depending on the degree of prominence of the alar lobule, the shape of the nasal tip, and the slope of the lateral walls, the Asian nose maybe grouped into 3 subtypes. The first group is characterized by a bulbous tip, prominent alar lobules that round off with broad alar bases, and a wide interalar angle. The second group is characterized by a better-defined tip, less prominent lobules, and a narrower interalar angle. In the final group, the lateral nasal walls slope down from a well-defined tip to the alar base in an almost straight plane, since the alar lobule prominence is minimal (yet still less tip projection and a wider interalar angle compared with Caucasians). Over 80% of Asians were classified into the first 2 groups.

Gruber and colleagues[43] also classified Asian American patients into 3 categories based on morphologic characteristics. In the first type, there is an overall vertical nasal height deficiency, a dorsal deficiency, and lack of adequate tip height. Although this results in a broader-appearing nose, there is not necessarily an absolute increase in alar or nasal bone width. In the second type, the patient also is deficient in overall vertical height but in addition exhibits an absolute increase in width of the nasal tip, nasal bones, and/or nasal base. Finally, in the third type, patients may have features of type 1 and type 2 noses, with the addition of a glabella deficiency, and in some cases the eyelids are anterior to the nasal root. The surgical management varies based on this classification, making the classification a helpful tool for the aesthetic analysis of the Asian nose:

Type 1: augmentation of dorsum and tip
Type 2: augmentation plus reduction of tip, nasal bone, and/or nasal base
Type 3: additional glabella augmentation

MIDDLE EASTERN RHINOPLASTY

The term Middle Eastern is used to describe a geographically and ethnically diverse population that includes people from countries in North Africa, the Arabian Peninsula, and Western Asia (ie, Egypt, Syria, Lebanon, Iraq, Jordan, Turkey, Saudi Arabia, and Iran). Rhinoplasty is one of the most commonly performed surgeries in this population, with a rate of rhinoplasty being 7 times more common in Iran than in the United States.[44] Although there are salient differences in nasal morphology and treatment goals among the diverse Middle Eastern patient population, certain generalizations have been made.

The skin in Middle Eastern patients is more variable than Caucasian patients. It is usually described as Fitzpatrick III to V and thought to be more sebaceous with thicker underlying soft tissue.[45] Although Rohrich and Mohan[45] have found thicker skin to be present in 90% of middle eastern noses, Daniel found this to be true in only 36% and cautioned against considering this to be a universal finding or the modification of the skin envelope in most patients.[46] In those with thicker skin, the effects of rhinoplasty may not be visible, and healing can be unpredictable. The nasal dorsum, both osseous and cartilaginous, is typically wider and more prominent in Middle Eastern patients.[45] Dorsal humps (osseocartilaginous > cartilage only > bony only) are common in Middle Eastern patients, and reduction of this is a common goal among Middle Eastern patients seeking rhinoplasty. Although the radix has commonly thought to be full and overprojected in Middle Eastern patients, this has surprisingly been shown to only be the case in 12% of patients.[46] The bony and middle nasal vaults are generally wider than in Caucasian patients, and an extreme width of the upper lateral cartilages at their scroll junction with the alar cartilages is a unique feature in Middle Eastern patients.[45,46]

The nasal tip is generally more bulbous appearing with a flattening of the domes relative to the anterior septal angle and drooping of the tip.[44–46] This results in an underprojected and under-rotated tip with an acute nasolabial angle and the illusion of increased nasal length.[47] A hyperactive depressor septi nasi also contributes to this nasal tip configuration and to a shorter philtrum length.[45] Ideally, the nasolabial angle in Middle Eastern patients is 90° to 95°.[48] The nasal base width is typically greater than that seen in Caucasians, with variable degrees of alar flaring present.[47]

The frequency and severity of nasal and facial asymmetry have been regarded by some to be more severe in Middle Eastern patients than in Caucasian patients. Nasal asymmetries exist in 82% of patients, and asymmetry of the osseocartilaginous vault is the rule rather than the exception in Middle Eastern patients.[45,46] Although no ideal standards of beauty have been described for the Middle Eastern nose, an improvement in nasal symmetry in this population is an essential treatment goal.

Although a broad understanding of the Middle Eastern nose is essential to approaching rhinoplasty in this patient population, the variability in phenotypes of the Middle Eastern nose cannot be overemphasized. A recent study examined the phenotypes of various Middle Eastern noses.[49] For example, the Egyptian nose is defined by wide nostrils, a sharp nasolabial angle, a rounded and broad tip, and wide dorsum with a small hump. Alternatively, the Levantine (Lebanon, Syria, Jordan) nose has a narrow yet arching dorsum and a fine nasal tip that is ptotic. The Turkish nose also has a plunging tip with inadequate projection, but a much wider nasal profile and prominent dorsal hump. Assyrians commonly have large noses with broad nasal tips, but with obtuse nasolabial angles. The noses of Kurds and Iraqis are also prominent with thick skin, while their Iranian neighbors frequently display less large but more crooked noses with thinner skin. All of these findings come with the caveat that historically there has been much mixing of races within these groups, and each individual must be considered in the context of his or her own anatomy and desires for change.

Aesthetic goals within the Middle Eastern patient population may also be variable. For example, women aged 25 to 55 years seek rhinoplasty for significantly improved definition of a nose that is perceived as too large.[46] Women under the age of 25 seek similar outcomes; however, they may prefer a natural look without evidence of surgical stigmata including pinched tips, retracted rims, nostril show, visible bossa, and inverted-V deformities. Rohrich and Mohan[45] also note that while male Middle Eastern patients similarly want improved definition and correction of a dorsal hump, they do not want an oversculpted look, unlike many female patients. As such, when combined with the morphologic variability of the nose, an individualized approach to patients of Middle Eastern descent is imperative.

SUMMARY

In the setting of increasing diversity observed among patients seeking rhinoplasty in the United States, facial plastic surgeons must understand nasal aesthetics in the context of race, ethnicity, and culture. A recent study has found an effect of observer race on social perception of nasal form before and after rhinoplasty.[50] The lack of clear aesthetic norms and ideal standards in non-Caucasian patients, in addition to the variation in nasal anatomy and morphology among races, can create a challenge in approaching ethnic rhinoplasty. Preoperative assessment of nasal and facial features that contribute to a nose that is unpleasing for a non-Caucasian patient cannot be based on neoclassical canons that have been used to detail ideal proportions, angles, and relationships between facial landmarks. Application of the ideal facial proportions and relationships in the Caucasian face to the ethnic rhinoplasty can result in loss of ethnic identity and patient dissatisfaction.

An essential goal of rhinoplasty is to achieve symmetry and improved definition without effacing ethnicity. An understanding of the anatomic and morphologic features that are common to different racial groups as described in this article can help a surgeon approach the non-Caucasian nose. Multiple other factors may also be taken into account when determining a patient's personal goals, including gender identity and its role in perception of nasal form, an issue not discussed herein.[51] Ultimately, a clear preoperative understanding of a patient's aesthetic goals, in the setting of his or her racial and ethnic identity, will maximize surgical outcomes and patient satisfaction.

DISCLOSURE

The authors have nothing to disclose.

REFERENCES

1. Vespa J, Medina L. Demographic turning points for the United States: population projections for 2020 to 2060. U.S. Census Bureau. Current Population Reports Web site. 2018. Avauilable at: https://www.census.gov/content/dam/Census/library/publications/2018/demo/P25_1144.pdf. Accessed May 10, 2019.

2. Sturm-O'Brien AK, Brissett AE, Brissett AE. Ethnic trends in facial plastic surgery. Facial Plast Surg 2010;26(2):69–74.

3. Broer PN, Levine SM, Juran S. Plastic surgery: quo vadis? Current trends and future projections of aesthetic plastic surgical procedures in the United States. Plast Reconstr Surg 2014;133(3):293e–302e.

4. Rohrich RJ, Bolden K. Ethnic rhinoplasty. Clin Plast Surg 2010;37(2):353–70.

5. Cobo R. Ethnic rhinoplasty. HNO 2018;66(1):6–14.

6. Bernstein L. Esthetics in rhinoplasty. Otolaryngol Clin North Am 1975;8(3): 705–15.

7. Leong SC, White PS. A comparison of aesthetic proportions between the healthy Caucasian nose and the aesthetic ideal. J Plast Reconstr Aesthet Surg 2006; 59(3):248–52.

8. Powell NHB. Proportions of the aesthetic face. New York: Theime-Stratton; 1984.

9. Millard DR. Adjuncts in augmentation mentoplasty and corrective rhinoplasty. Plast Reconstr Surg 1965;36:48–61.

10. Papel ID. Facial plastic and reconstructive surgery. New York: Thieme; 2016.

11. Crumley RL, Lanser M. Quantitative analysis of nasal tip projection. Laryngoscope 1988;98(2):202–8.

12. Bueller H. Ideal facial relationships and goals. Facial Plast Surg 2018;34(5): 458–65.

13. Porter JP, Olson KL. Analysis of the African American female nose. Plast Reconstr Surg 2003;111(2):620–6 [discussion: 627–8].

14. Milgrim LM, Lawson W, Cohen AF. Anthropometric analysis of the female Latino nose. Revised aesthetic concepts and their surgical implications. Arch Otolaryngol Head Neck Surg 1996;122(10):1079–86.

15. Mehta N, Srivastava RK. The Indian nose: an anthropometric analysis. J Plast Reconstr Aesthet Surg 2017;70(10):1472–82.

16. Aung SC, Foo CL, Lee ST. Three dimensional laser scan assessment of the Oriental nose with a new classification of Oriental nasal types. Br J Plast Surg 2000; 53(2):109–16.

17. Rhee SC. Differences between Caucasian and Asian attractive faces. Skin Res Technol 2018;24(1):73–9.

18. Patel AD, Kridel RW. African-American rhinoplasty. Facial Plast Surg 2010;26(2): 131–41.

19. Davis RE. Rhinoplasty and concepts of facial beauty. Facial Plast Surg 2006; 22(3):198–203.

20. Farkas LG, Kolar JC, Munro IR. Geography of the nose: a morphometric study. Aesthetic Plast Surg 1986;10(4):191–223.

21. Leach J. Aesthetics and the Hispanic rhinoplasty. Laryngoscope 2002;112(11): 1903–16.

22. Baker H, Krause C. Update on the negroid nose: an anatomic and anthropometric analysis. St Louis (MO): CV Mosby and Company; 1984.

23. Ofodile FA, Bokhari FJ, Ellis C. The black American nose. Ann Plast Surg 1993; 31(3):209–18 [discussion: 218–9].

24. Boyette JR, Stucker FJ. African American rhinoplasty. Facial Plast Surg Clin North Am 2014;22(3):379–93.

25. Rohrich RJ, Muzaffar AR. Rhinoplasty in the African-American patient. Plast Reconstr Surg 2003;111(3):1322–39 [discussion: 1340–1].

26. Peng GL, Nassif PS. Rhinoplasty in the African American patient: anatomic considerations and technical pearls. Clin Plast Surg 2016;43(1):255–64.

27. Ofodile FA, James EA. Anatomy of alar cartilages in blacks. Plast Reconstr Surg 1997;100(3):699–703.

28. Chike-Obi CJ, Boahene K, Bullocks JM, et al. Tip nuances for the nose of African descent. Facial Plast Surg 2012;28(2):194–201.

29. Ofodile FA, Bokhari F. The African-American nose: part II. Ann Plast Surg 1995; 34(2):123–9.

30. Porter JP. The average African American male face: an anthropometric analysis. Arch Facial Plast Surg 2004;6(2):78–81.

31. Ofodile FA. Nasal bones and pyriform apertures in blacks. Ann Plast Surg 1994; 32(1):21–6.

32. Cobo R. Hispanic/Mestizo rhinoplasty. Facial Plast Surg Clin North Am 2010; 18(1):173–88.

33. Ortiz-Monasterio F, Olmedo A. Rhinoplasty on the mestizo nose. Clin Plast Surg 1977;4(1):89–102.

34. Cobo R. Facial aesthetic surgery with emphasis on rhinoplasty in the Hispanic patient. Curr Opin Otolaryngol Head Neck Surg 2008;16(4):369–75.

35. Patel AD, Kridel RW. Hispanic-American rhinoplasty. Facial Plast Surg 2010; 26(2):142–53.

36. Higuera S, Hatef DA, Stal S. Rhinoplasty in the Hispanic patient. Semin Plast Surg 2009;23(3):207–14.

37. Daniel RK. Hispanic rhinoplasty in the United States, with emphasis on the Mexican American nose. Plast Reconstr Surg 2003;112(1):244–56 [discussion: 257–8].

38. Tansatit T, Moon HJ, Rungsawang C, et al. Safe planes for injection rhinoplasty: a histological analysis of midline longitudinal sections of the Asian nose. Aesthetic Plast Surg 2016;40(2):236–44.

39. Jang YJ, Alfanta EM. Rhinoplasty in the Asian nose. Facial Plast Surg Clin North Am 2014;22(3):357–77.

40. Moon KC, Han SK. Surgical anatomy of the Asian nose. Facial Plast Surg Clin North Am 2018;26(3):259–68.

41. Jin HR, Won TB. Rhinoplasty in the Asian patient. Clin Plast Surg 2016;43(1): 265–79.

42. Jang YJ, Yu MS. Rhinoplasty for the Asian nose. Facial Plast Surg 2010;26(2): 93–101.

43. Gruber R, Kuang A, Kahn D. Asian-American rhinoplasty. Aesthet Surg J 2004; 24(5):423–30.

44. Pourdanesh F, Dehghani N, Azarsina M, et al. Pattern of odontogenic infections at a tertiary hospital in tehran, iran: a 10-year retrospective study of 310 patients. J Dent 2013;10(4):319–28.

45. Rohrich RJ, Mohan R. Middle eastern rhinoplasty: update. Plast Reconstr Surg Glob Open 2018;6(12):e1984.

46. Daniel RK. Middle Eastern rhinoplasty: anatomy, aesthetics, and surgical planning. Facial Plast Surg 2010;26(2):110–8.

47. Azizzadeh B, Mashkevich G. Middle Eastern rhinoplasty. Facial Plast Surg Clin North Am 2010;18(1):201–6.

48. Sajjadian A. Rhinoplasty in Middle Eastern patients. Clin Plast Surg 2016;43(1): 281–94.

49. Niechajev I. Noses of the Middle East: variety of phenotypes and surgical approaches. J Craniofac Surg 2016;27(7):1700–6.

50. Darrach H, Ishii LE, Liao D, et al. Assessment of the Influence of "Other-Race Effect" on visual attention and perception of attractiveness before and after rhinoplasty. JAMA Facial Plast Surg 2019;21(2):96–102.
51. Nuyen B, Kandathil CK, Saltychev M, et al. Social perception of the nasal dorsal contour in male rhinoplasty. JAMA Facial Plast Surg 2019. https://doi.org/10.1001/jamafacial.2019.0321.

How You See Yourself
Cultural Considerations and Self-Image for Rhinoplasty Patients

Anisha R. Kumar, MD, Lisa E. Ishii, MD, MHS*

KEYWORDS

- Anthropology • Ideal beauty • Self-image • Stereotype

KEY POINTS

- Patient ethnicity presents the unique challenge in facial plastic surgery of incorporating individual preference while maintaining certain physical characteristics.
- Motivations of pursuing ethnic-sensitive rhinoplasty include achieving the perceived ideal of anatomic beauty constructed within an ethnic community and escaping negative stereotypes as suggested by certain physical characteristics.
- It is important to recognize the implications of ethnic-sensitive rhinoplasty, such as potentially of reinforcing the construction and implications of stereotypes and the effects on self-image.

INTRODUCTION

The concepts of race and ethnicity are often used interchangeably in medicine. Although race has been used to signify a group of individuals with similar physical characteristics secondary to shared genetic ancestry, in this article, the authors will use ethnicity to signify a category of individuals with similar physical characteristics who also have a shared history, language, heritage, or customs. Culture refers to the system of shared beliefs, customs, values, and behaviors employed by members of a group.

In the realm of facial plastic and reconstructive surgery, patient ethnicity presents the unique challenge of incorporating individual preference while maintaining certain physical characteristics. Furthermore, the psychosocial influences that drive patients of different ethnicities vary, and therefore this article seeks to elucidate an understanding of the cultural considerations and implications of facial cosmetic surgery that is crucial for surgeons.

Department of Otolaryngology–Head and Neck Surgery, The Johns Hopkins University School of Medicine, Johns Hopkins Outpatient Center, 601 North Caroline Street, Baltimore, MD 21287, USA
* Corresponding author.
E-mail address: learnes2@jhmi.edu

Otolaryngol Clin N Am 53 (2020) 209–212
https://doi.org/10.1016/j.otc.2019.12.002
0030-6665/20/© 2019 Elsevier Inc. All rights reserved.

oto.theclinics.com

CONTENT
Cultural and Institutional Forces as Motivation

There is little research on the perception of rhinoplasty among various ethnic groups. However, because the well-described concept of the other race effect, it has been extrapolated that members of a certain racial group have greater discernment in assessing facial beauty in their community and therefore perceptions of rhinoplasty.[1]

To achieve the ideal

According to sociocultural theory, people internalize the standards of beauty according to their context of community. With specific standards of beauty in a cultural community, a pervasive motivation of pursuing ethnic sensitive surgery is to achieve the perceived ideal of anatomic beauty. As certain groups historically have been described as having distinct physical characteristics (eg, the differences in dorsum, projection, and rotation among African, Asian, and white noses), patients want to seek the ideal of nasal anatomy within the range of characteristic that is biologically prevalent and plausible for their racial group, in order to still maintain physical identification with that group.[2] However, the culturally constructed anatomic ideal nose is a nuanced concept that reflects not only present-day global influence but also historic notions. Aquino[3] argues that the beauty standards for East Asians are constructed from interplay between cultural imperialism and cultural nationalism, suggesting an influence of westernization in Asia but also a desire to maintain anatomy features of the historically valued East Asian conceptualization of beauty.

Furthermore, because of this nuanced interplay of influential factors, the specific ideals of beauty of the nose vary greatly among ethnic groups. In the Latino culture, the concept of mestizo reflects a historic mix of European and Native American features that results in the conceptualized ideal external nose having increased tip definition and projection.[4] For example, in an ethnographic study done in Venezuela, community members preferred to have decreased nasal width, as this was seen to be less consistent with the mestizo ideal and more suggestive of an association with blackness ancestrally.[5] Additionally, the culturally specific ideal nose continues to support the notion of the layered influences of westernization and of historic beauty standards. Qualitative research has shown that the East Asian ideal nose has a chiseled appearance and prominent nasal bridge,[6] while the African ideal nose also a prominent nasal bridge but also reduced nasal width.[7]

Although there are variations in the ideal nose among ethnic groups, is there commonality in what drives individuals to pursue these ideals? Across different communities in the present day and historically, the pursuit of ideal beauty has been an indication of socioeconomic status. For example, in twentieth century Austria and Germany, the presence of nasal deformity was one ideal for males because it was suggestive of facial injury during the sport of fencing, thus indicative of the participant's social status needed to in order to participate in such activities.[8] Similarly, the ability to undergo cosmetic surgery is viewed as an elite symbol for women in Japan and Korea; however, cosmetic surgery in China is viewed in more a nuanced way, not only as an elite symbol but also as a transformation from the communist woman to the progressive Westernized liberal.[3]

Finally, in spite of some similarity in motivation for facial cosmetic surgery, there are subtle differences in the implications of pursuing the ideal for anatomy beauty among racial groups. In assessing the population of casual observers in the United States, rhinoplasty was associated with more perceived attractiveness, success, and health.[9] Furthermore, in a cross-country comparison between the United States and India, although increasing perceived attractiveness with facelift surgery was valued in both societies, the desire to reduce perceived age through this cosmetic intervention was only significantly valued in the United States but not India, theorized to reflect that reduction in age in a component of the cultural construct of beauty in the United States but not necessarily in other cultures (Kumar AR, Ishii M, Papel I, et al. Perception and valuation of rhytidectomy among different racial groups. Facial Plastic Surgery 2019, under review.). Furthermore, in certain racial groups, the goal of achieving the ideal beauty standard has specific implications in social perceptions; ethnographic research has revealed that among certain South Asian, Middle Eastern, and East Asian communities, patients associated facial cosmetic surgery as an way to improve prospects of marriage.[3,8]

To escape stereotypes

Although the desire to achieve the ideal beauty standard has been a long-standing reason for the prevalence of rhinoplasty among different ethnic groups, the desire to escape negative stereotypes as suggested by certain physical characteristics has also been a driving factor. Ethnographic research in East Asian communities suggests that the members believe the stereotypical flat nasal dorsum implied that one was passive and dull, therefore leading to decreased sociability.[10] Therefore, ethnic rhinoplasty is seen as a mechanism of improving one's perceived personality and potentially even increasing social interaction. In communities in Venezuela, a wide nasal width contributes to racial discrimination, even teasing in schools, for an association with blackness.[5] Thus in this situation, ethnic rhinoplasty is an opportunity to distance oneself from certain racial groups and possibly even redefine one's own racial association. Furthermore, it is important to recognize that by pursuing rhinoplasty to avoid certain stereotypes based on external nasal anatomy, ethnic groups are inadvertently reinforcing the construction and implications of these stereotypes. The concerning aspect of this irony is that the reinforcing of ethnocentric characteristics may ultimately contribute to negatively impacting self-image of the patients who chose this procedure for the opposite result.[6] Nonetheless, the implication of being able to navigate stereotypes through alteration of the external nose is that there is fluidity in the concept of identity.

Self-Image of Ethnic Rhinoplasty Patients

In addition to the cultural influences on ethnic rhinoplasty patients, it is equally as important to understand the individual motivation and perspective of each patient in order to better craft treatment options and manage expectations.

A distinct difference among different ethnic groups is the anatomic focus on self-image. The prospective study by Lee[11] showed considerable gender and ethnic difference in self-image and attitude toward cosmetic procedures; white female participants were predominantly focused on whole-body appearance and satisfaction while Asian female participants focused on facial appearance, with concern over eye and nose. These differences are important not only for to manage patient expectations but also for to develop marketing strategies to different ethnic groups to address their distinct concerns about self-image.

Furthermore, in assessing self-image and personal motivations for pursuing ethnic rhinoplasty, it is important to note the prevalence of body dysmorphic disorder (BDD) among the population of cosmetic surgery patients. In an analysis at 3 academic centers in the United States, 13.1% of patients presenting to clinic for facial cosmetic concerns screened positive for BDD.[12] Although little research has been done on the prevalence of BDD among different ethnic groups pursuing cosmetic facial surgery, the multifactorial motivation of cultural ideals and motivation of targeted improvement in self-image may result in a higher incidence of BDD among patients who undergo ethnic-sensitive surgery, and this should be further explored in each physician-patient interaction.

SUMMARY

With the growth and nuances of ethnic-sensitive rhinoplasty, an understanding of the cultural and institutional motivations will reveal the desire to achieve the ideal beauty standard for a certain group and the drive to navigate stereotypes. However, in the midst of these motivations, it is important to acknowledge the impact of rhinoplasty on the self-image of the ethnic patient. Additionally, there are ethical considerations in ethnic-sensitive rhinoplasty including the medicalization of racial features and the increased agency of racial minorities and women achieved through this intervention. Ultimately, this article seeks to highlight the importance of surgeons developing cross-cultural sensitivity and an understanding of cultural norms, in addition to managing the patient's expectation of ethnic rhinoplasty.[8] Over time, the motivation for ethnic sensitive rhinoplasty will continue to evolve as the homogeneity of racial groups decreases.

DISCLOSURE

The authors have nothing to disclose.

REFERENCES

1. Darrach H, Ishii LE, Liao D, et al. Assessment of the influence of "other-race effect" on visual attention and perception of attractiveness before and after rhinoplasty. JAMA Facial Plast Surg 2019;21(2):96–102.
2. Weeks DM, Thomas RJ. Beauty in a multicultural world. Facial Plast Surg Clin North Am 2014;22(3):337–41.
3. Aquino YSJ. Borrowed beauty? Understanding identity in Asian facial cosmetic surgery. Med Health Care Philos 2016. https://doi.org/10.1007/s11019-016-9699-0.
4. Cobo R. Rhinoplaty in Latino patients. Clin Plast Surg 2016;43(1):237–54.
5. Gulbas L. Embodying racism: race, rhinoplasty, and self-esteem in Venezuela. Qual Health Res 2013;23(3):326–35.
6. Kaw E. Medicalization of racial features: Asian American women and cosmetic surgery. Med Anthropol Q 1993;7(1):74–89.
7. Slupchynskyj O, Gieniusz M. Rhinoplasty for African American patients. JAMA Facial Plast Surg 2008;10(4):232–6.
8. Rowe-Jones J. Facial aesthetic surgical goals in patients of difference cultures. Facial Plast Surg Clin North Am 2014;22(3):343–8.
9. Nellis J, Ishii M, Bater K, et al. Association of rhinoplasty with perceived attractiveness, success, and overall health. JAMA Facial Plast Surg 2018;20(2):97–102.
10. Kaw E. Medicalization of Racial Features: Asian American Women and Cosmetic Surgery. Medical Anthropology Quarterly 1993;7(1):74–89.
11. Lee M. Body satisfaction and attitudes towards cosmetic surgical vs. nonsurgical procedures. Internal Journal of Humanities and Social Science 2016;6(10):34–9.
12. Joseph A, Ishii LE, Joseph SS, et al. Prevalance of body dysmorphic disorder and surgeon diagnostic accuracy in facial plastic and occuloplastic clinics. JAMA Facial Plast Surg 2017;19(4):269–74.

Finesse in Caucasian Endonasal Rhinoplasty
The S.O.F.T. Concept

Holger G. Gassner, MD[a,b],*

KEYWORDS

- Endonasal rhinoplasty • Ethnic rhinoplasty • Caucasian rhinoplasty
- Endonasal complete release approach • S.O.F.T. concept • Soft nasal tip
- Soft tissue sanctuaries • Preseptal deformation zone

KEY POINTS

- Anatomic characteristics of the Caucasian nose include a thin skin–soft tissue envelope; limited soft tissue reserve; high dorsum; strong cartilaginous framework; and narrow, elliptical nasal inlets.
- The S.O.F.T. (surgery and ongoing care free of trauma) concept is presented as a holistic approach to endonasal Caucasian rhinoplasty. It consists of 7 cardinal principles: (1) perform an endonasal operation, (2) save the soft tissue sanctuaries, (3) restructure the lower lateral cartilages — as foreseen by nature, (4) limit to 4 autologous graft types, (5) conserve anatomic structures within their habitats, (6) preserve all turbinate soft tissue, and (7) apply minimally invasive techniques.
- Innovations include the endonasal complete release approach, natural recontouring of the lower lateral cartilages, the stairstep graft for correction of the nasal valve, the foundation graft for correction of the secondary cleft deformity, free diced cartilage in dermis (DCID) grafts to address skin compromise in revisional scenarios, the description of defined soft tissue sanctuaries (cartilage-void zones) and of the preseptal deformation zone (compartment designed to absorb head-on trauma) of the nose.
- Alternatives to the following methods are presented: the tongue-in-groove maneuver, the L-strut concept, liberal costal cartilage grafting, cartilage-weakening techniques, tip grafting, alar rim grafting, and reduction/destruction of turbinate submucosa.
- A didactic concept is presented that streamlines the surgical options available and facilitates inclusion of the endonasal operation in any established rhinoplasty practice.

INTRODUCTION

The Caucasian nose features a unique set of anatomic characteristics. These characteristics include:

a Finesse Center for Facial Plastic Surgery Regensburg, Regensburg, Germany; b Faculty of Medicine, University of Regensburg, Regensburg, Germany
* Froehliche – Tuerken – Strasse 8, Regensburg 93047, Germany.
E-mail address: info@drgassner.eu

Otolaryngol Clin N Am 53 (2020) 213–235
https://doi.org/10.1016/j.otc.2019.12.006
0030-6665/20/© 2019 Elsevier Inc. All rights reserved.

- A thin skin–soft tissue envelope requiring special attention to achieve smooth postsurgical contours
- A narrow and prominent nasal bridge frequently calling for reductive techniques
- An important contribution of the cartilaginous skeleton to overall structural support, requiring stable skeletal support grafts when deficiencies are present
- A narrow, elliptical nasal inlet predisposing to nasal valve obstruction
- Greater susceptibility of the skin to swelling and bruising, calling for particularly gentle surgical techniques
- A smaller reserve of cartilage-void zones, reducing the residual deformation capacity after surgical intervention and calling for conservative grafting in order to maintain a soft-feeling nasal tip

Important influences have been instrumental in the development of the S.O.F.T. (surgery and ongoing care free of trauma) concept:

- The strict demands of my mentors Eugene Kern to preserve endonasal physiology, and David Sherris and Wayne Larrabee to maximize gentle soft tissue handling[1–4]
- The minimal invasive endonasal approaches of Norman Pastorek
- The open-structure concept of Johnson and Toriumi[1]
- The need to provide a simplified didactic concept for fellows
- The patients' requests to obtain a naturally appearing, beautiful outcome; to maintain a natural soft touch to the nasal tip; and to experience easy and short recovery with early nasal airway patency

Moreover, ongoing long-term patient interviews have allowed a better understanding of patient expectations. This feedback results in continuous adaptions to clinical and surgical care and has influenced the evolution of the S.O.F.T. concept over the past decade. It has proved successful in my personal experience of more than 2000 endonasal rhinoplasties, about half of them revisions. The concept commands 7 objectives and 7 corresponding principles.

The 7 objectives of the S.O.F.T. concept are:

1. Achieve a naturally beautiful look.
2. Maintain a soft-feeling nasal tip.
3. Conserve the anatomic configuration of the nose as foreseen by nature.
4. Provide a coherent and structured didactic concept.
5. Reduce risk for and extent of revisional surgery.
6. Preserve endonasal physiologic function.
7. Provide for expedited and comfortable recovery.

CONTENT
The S.O.F.T. Concept in Endonasal Rhinoplasty

This article presents a stand-alone concept for endonasal rhinoplasty. By no means does it compete with, let alone criticize, the open approach or other endonasal concepts. The author holds the work of Dean Toriumi and other excellent surgeons committed to the open approach in the highest regard. The S.O.F.T. concept integrates important aspects of the open structure concepts and could never have been developed without the ingenious contributions of the pioneers of open structure rhinoplasty. It is emphasized that the concepts of the endonasal and the open operations are regarded as completely separate entities.

Data presented were extracted from a rhinoplasty outcome database that was created with approval of the Institutional Review Board of the Faculty of Medicine,

University of Regensburg. Where needed, additional informed consent was obtained from patients for presentation of identifiable data and images.

The 7 S.O.F.T. concept objectives as listed earlier are achieved by applying the following, corresponding 7 cardinal principles:

1. Perform an endonasal operation.
2. Save the soft tissue sanctuaries.
3. Restructure the lower lateral cartilages (LLCs) to look natural.
4. Limit to 4 autologous graft types.
5. Conserve anatomic structures within their habitats.
6. Preserve of all the turbinate soft tissue.
7. Apply minimally invasive techniques.

These principles give structure to the following discussion.

First cardinal principle: perform an endonasal operation
Endonasal versus open approach Data from 291 patients of the Regensburg Rhinoplasty Database were analyzed to compare functional and cosmetic outcomes from a time when the author performed exclusively open rhinoplasty with a time when the author performed exclusively endonasal operations. A detailed discussion of these data would exceed the scope of this report and will be presented in a future publication. Briefly, **Fig. 1** shows that mean cosmetic outcome, as assessed by lay and expert

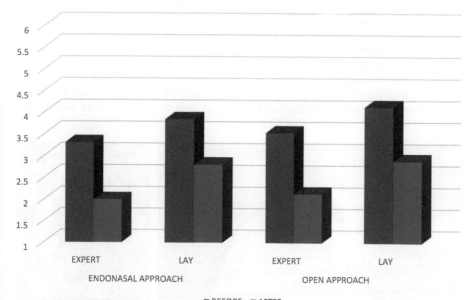

Fig. 1. Data comparing cosmetic outcome after open versus endonasal rhinoplasty. The data for open and endonasal rhinoplasty were obtained from phases in the author's career when he performed almost exclusively open endonasal operations. Thus, patient demographics and severity of deformity are comparable between the two groups. No operator-dependent confounding factors are present. Results were obtained by blinded assessment of cosmetic outcome by an expert and a lay panel of 3 evaluators. Assessment was performed on a 6-cm visual analog scale with 1 being ideal and 6 being a very poor outcome. For both expert and lay evaluations, no significant or relevant differences between the endonasal and the open operation were present.

panel evaluations of standardized photographs, was equal between the endonasal and the open operations. The functional data, based on the Nasal Obstruction Symptom Evaluation (NOSE) instrument questionnaire, show equal outcomes as well. All relevant confounding parameters, such as demographic data and proportion of revisional surgery, were comparable between the two groups. Of note, the study populations included complex congenital and revisional cases including costal cartilage transfer.

These data, as well as experience with managing a revision-heavy endonasal rhinoplasty practice for about a decade, suggest that the endonasal and the open operations differ in many important aspects but share equivalent potency and outcomes. Other large series also show equivalent outcomes when eras of endonasal and open operations are compared.[5,6]

Endonasal operation: basics and principles The cartilaginous skeleton of the nose maintains its three-dimensional form to a large degree by the tension-banding effects of the overlying soft tissue. Release of these forces unmasks a large number of deformities. This observation may explain the inflation of descriptions of corrective open suture and grafting maneuvers, many of which are likely the result of correcting previously masked skeletal irregularities. **Fig. 2** shows this effect.

With the application of endonasal approaches, surface contour rather than skeletal irregularities determines the selection of corrective maneuvers. However, this does not imply that endonasal rhinoplasty is to be regarded as a subtraction-addition procedure. On the contrary, it is emphasized that the endonasal S.O.F.T. concept does not predominantly rely on contour grafting. Endonasal structural grafting and natural-looking recontouring of the skeletal framework are pursued in order to achieve ideal shape. When minor contour irregularities (1 mm or less) remain, these are camouflaged with small volumes of shaved or diced cartilage and/or fascial grafts.

Grafting and suture techniques behave profoundly differently when applied endonasally. This difference is highlighted by the fact that an intraoperative switch from

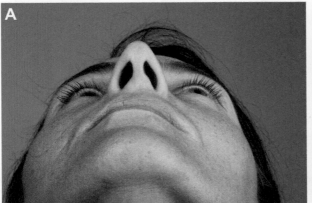 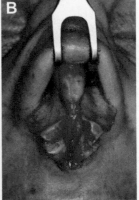

Fig. 2. (*A*) Preoperative image shows a minimal left-sided bulge of the columellar base, which can be corrected with limited retrograde partial undermining of the columella, potentially scoring of the left medial crus, resection of interpedal soft tissue, and placement of a transcolumellar mattress suture. (*B*) After completion of an open approach, extensive irregularities of the medial crura are unmasked bilaterally. This crumbling appearance lends itself to placement of a stenting graft along the length of the medial crura.

endonasal to the open approach is infrequently described or lectured about. Simply, the 2 approaches cannot be applied interchangeably: the operation changes its character with the approach. The dynamics and elasticity of the tip-columellar complex alone are representative of these diverging scenarios. The principles of tip management described herein falter when the recoil of the infratip complex is lost.

Because the procedure changes its character so profoundly, it is suggested to use the term endonasal versus open operation rather than approach. It is also suggested that it suits the opposite character of these different operations better if they are discussed in dedicated segments at conferences and courses.

The endonasal operation forms the foundation of the S.O.F.T. concept for the following reasons:

1. Preservation of the fibrous network of the infratip lobule and membranous septum provides stable elastic recoil of the mesial crura, which is consecutively transmitted to the domal segments and lateral crura. This elasticity allows for maintenance of softness and provides an important hinge mechanism for the lateral crural cartilage. Moreover, the nose is better protected against trauma when this preseptal deformation zone (described later) is preserved.
2. Preservation of the columellar neurovascular bundles maintains the only gravity-accentuated venous and lymphatic drainage system of the nose. Moreover, the neurovascular innervation of the nasal tip skin is maintained. Thus, postoperative edema should be reduced and the skin may be protected from long-term neurovascular denervation atrophy.
3. Extensive tissue stretch (eg, with cleft nose correction) is well tolerated by an anatomically intact columellar complex and allows for effective, low-risk projection of the nasal tip, even in difficult scenarios.
4. Immediate readaption of the skin–soft tissue envelope allows for excellent continuous intraoperative assessment of contour changes.
5. Exposure of the wound surfaces of the dorsal flap to ambient air and desiccation trauma is reduced, which is hypothesized to reduce edema and to enhance postoperative recovery.

The endonasal operation is highly versatile. The following represent the spectrum of routinely used approaches in my practice:

1. Intercartilaginous incision approach
2. Transcartilaginous incision approach
3. Transvestibular approach of Fuleihan[7]
4. Combined intercartilaginous and hemitransfixion incision approach
5. Delivery approach
6. Endonasal complete release (ECR) approach

The endonasal operation is erroneously perceived to be limited by narrower exposure and more restricted ability to modify the nasal tip. Some of these limitations may, to some degree depending on operator expertise, be associated with the longer-established approaches (1–5). With the description of the ECR approach (6), perceived limitations of the endonasal approach can be eliminated. The ECR opens the spectrum of indications to include the most challenging revisional and congenital scenarios. It was first performed in 2009 and was published in 2013 with a review of 100 consecutive cases.[8] From 01/2009 until 12/2018, a total of 901 ECR approaches were completed, accounting for approximately half of the 1815 endonasal operations performed during that period.

Exposure It is often argued that the endonasal operation is associated with limited lateral exposure. Lateral limitation of endonasal exposure is a misconception. There is no anatomic structure that is released with the open operation that restricts lateral access. Complete lateral extension of the intercartilaginous incision can open a very wide field with exposure all the way over the nasofacial crease and up to the infraorbital foramen. Lateral Piezo osteotomy, for instance, can in principle be completed under direct visualization with wide exposure, as shown in **Fig. 3**.

Although wide lateral exposure can be achieved, it is stressed that selection of the least extensive endonasal approach forms an integral element of the S.O.F.T. concept: access is generated that is broad enough to allow for precise execution of all required maneuvers. Broad lateral expansion to accommodate larger instruments such as the Piezotome is avoided when smaller alternative instruments permit the same effect through a more limited approach. At present, I largely reserve the use of the Piezotome for paramedian osteotomies, dorsal contouring, and congenital deformities, and rely on small conventional straight osteotomes for deep straight lateral osteotomies.

The middle third may be widely exposed by connecting an intercartilaginous with a hemitransfixion incision. Structural reconstruction of the middle third is easily achieved through this exposure, as shown in **Fig. 4**.

Endonasal exposure of the septal space is not limited. When needed, the upper lateral cartilages are released. Emphasis is placed on preserving residual septal cartilage and correcting deformities and deficiencies in the least intrusive manner.

The nasal tip can be widely exposed with the delivery technique. When this is insufficient, exposure can be escalated with use of the ECR.

The endonasal complete release approach The ECR has evolved from the observation that the interdomal suture applied through the delivery approach has a tendency to medialize the scroll region and thus negatively affect nasal valve function.

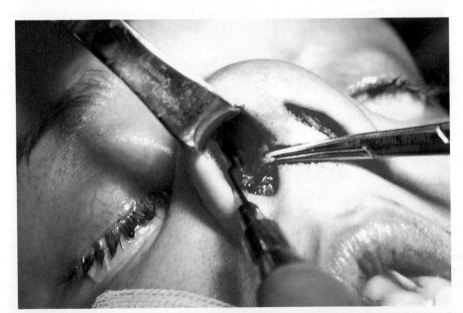

Fig. 3. Lateral extension of the endonasal operation is not limited. When required, this dissection can be continued across the midface to visualize the infraorbital foramen.

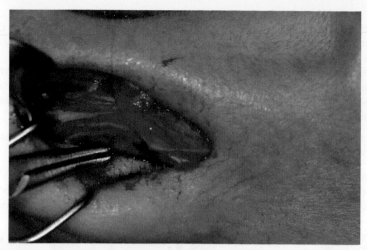

Fig. 4. Endonasal approaches allow for wide exposure, complete analysis, modification, and reconstruction of the middle third. Suture fixation of spreader-flaps is shown.

Moreover, deprojection sometimes requires shortening of the lateral crus. To avoid transecting the lateral crus in such scenarios, bilaminar release of the lateral crus allows alteration of the dome position by medial or lateral steal and advancement without transection. However, complete release weakens the lateral crus and necessitates the placement of an alar strut graft. The collateral beneficial effects of the maneuvers listed earlier include:

- Improvement of nasal valve function
- Reorientation of the lateral crus
- Control over the soft triangle and alar rim
- Control over nasal tip width and shape

In detail, the ECR is performed as follows. A marginal incision is extended into a paracolumellar incision of varying length (may be extended all the way to the columellar base). In order to optimize septal and dorsal access, an intercartilaginous incision is frequently placed and joined with a right hemitransfixion incision.

Bilaminar supraperichondrial dissection releases the lateral crus and allows identification and transection of the piriform ligament. It is important to recognize that the piriform ligament represents an extension of the lateral crus that fuses with the piriform crest. The domal angle is completely freed and the medial crus developed as far as required. This procedure results in complete release of the lateral crus. Now the following maneuvers can be pursued:

1. The domal angle may be modified, or translocated with a medial or lateral crural steal maneuver. When a new domal angle is created with scoring and suture techniques, the old domal angle is stented with an alar strut graft and potentially through fine scoring. The ability to modify the shape and position of the dome is almost unlimited in all dimensions because the completely released lateral crus is free of all soft tissue restrictions. Its curve, shape, and tension are recreated as foreseen by nature; contour (eg, shield) grafts are not needed.
2. A lateral crural strut graft is routinely placed when the lateral crus has been released. This graft reinforces the nasal valve at its most critical region, referred to as the point of first contact on collapse. As a result, nasal valve function is enhanced or valve dysfunction prevented.

3. Adaptions of the shape of the lateral crural strut graft, including its inferior confines and control over the angular orientation of the grafted lateral crus, allow for very powerful correction of alar retraction and deformities of the soft triangle.
4. The freely mobile and stented lateral crus is usually transposed into a more horizontal position, placed and, if needed, fixated in a generously dissected pocket over the piriform crest. This technique allows correction of deformities associated with alar malposition and is applied in a large proportion of cases.

Fig. 5 shows representative surgical steps of an ECR. See the original description and online video material for more details.[9]

Second cardinal principle: save the soft tissue sanctuaries

Besides cosmesis and airway, the tactile feedback of the nose is important for the patient's quality of life. The nose is among the most projected and most commonly

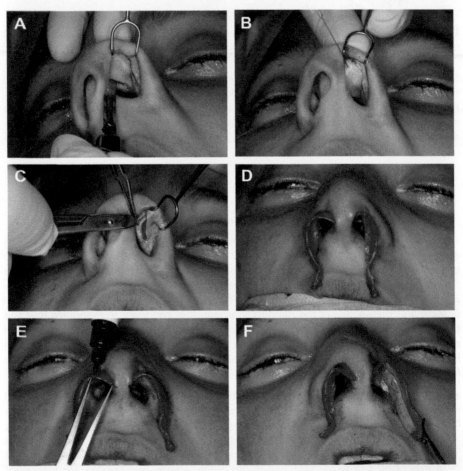

Fig. 5. (*A–F*) The steps of an ECR approach. (*A*) After placement of an intercartilaginous and a marginal incision, (*B*) hydrodissection and (*C*) gentle dissection of the vestibular skin are pursued. (*D*) After bilaminar release and transection of the piriform ligament, the lower lateral cartilages (LLCs) are delivered. (*E*) Measurements allow for (*F*) precise recontouring of the LLC by means of medial crural steal, placement of interdomal and intradomal sutures, and fixation of alar strut grafts.

touched features of the face. A natural softness of the face and nose is likely key in forming a positive body image both of the patient and for the patient's partner. Maintaining a soft nasal tip is therefore essential in achieving a natural rhinoplasty outcome.

The Soft Tissue Sanctuaries of the Nose

The natural softness of the human nose is mediated by 4 cartilage-free zones, as shown in **Fig. 6**A:

1. The membranous septum
2. The interdomal space
3. The soft triangles
4. The fibromuscular soft tissues of the ala

The term soft tissue sanctuaries describes these cartilage-free zones, and the S.O.F.T. concept stipulates their preservation.

The membranous septum and the interdomal space form part of an important functional entity, the preseptal deformation zone, which is particularly important

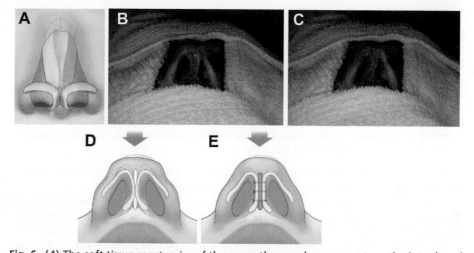

Fig. 6. (A) The soft tissue sanctuaries of the nose: the membranous septum, the interdomal space, the soft triangles, and the fibromuscular tissues of the ala mediate the naturally soft texture of the human nose. The S.O.F.T. concept stipulates preservation of these cartilage-void zones. (B) Partial dissection of the preseptal deformation zone: residual soft tissue attachments maintain the tension-banding effects that keep the intercrural space and provide elastic recoil to the important central compartment. (C) After violation of 2 important soft tissue sanctuaries (ie, the membranous septum and the interdomal space), the central compartment loses its elastic recoil, structural support diminishes, and the intercrural space is lost. Consequently, intercrural grafting becomes necessary in surgical practice. Linear beam grafting (with a columellar strut or the like) does not provide for the elasticity that is maintained by the mechanisms of curved beam recoil, closed space decompression, and interconnective fiber recoil, as described in the text. (D) The preseptal deformation zone allows for effective mitigation of head-on shock by various mechanisms, including bending of the medial crura, posterior advancement of the columella relative to the caudal septum, stretching of the tension-banding system, and increase in intracompartmental pressure. (E) Central compartment dissection and grafting reduces the ability of the medial crura to recoil and relax, renders the central soft tissue compartment firmer, and can eliminate the ability of the columella-tip complex to advance posteriorly relative to the septum, when a tongue-in-groove technique is used.

in mediating tip softness in the central compartment. **Fig. 6**B to D show the concept.

The preseptal deformation zone

Closely related to tip softness, and just as important, is the ability of the nose to mitigate trauma. The mechanisms lending softness to the tip are similar, but not identical, to those designed to defuse head-on shock and therefore warrant separate consideration. The shock-absorbing mechanisms of the nose are provided by a defined anatomic space. This space is confined superiorly by the caudal end of the septum and its virtual anterior extension, posteriorly by the anterior nasal spine, inferiorly by the skin coverage of the columella and infratip lobule, and anteriorly by the skin of the tip. This anatomic area can be thought of as the preseptal deformation zone. It contains the preseptal soft tissues up to the interdomal space, paired curved cartilaginous beams (from the medial crural footplate to the domal angle), and named and unnamed ligamentous interconnections lending a tension-banding effect to these skeletal structures. **Fig. 6**D, E show the divergent response of the preseptal deformation zone to head-on shock in the preserved and in the dissected/grafted state.

Head-on shock is absorbed in 4 ways:

1. The curved cartilaginous beams of the medial crura and domes deform by accentuating their natural curvature and recoil to their original state.
2. The network of fibrous and ligamentous soft tissue interconnections stretches and relaxes to its original state.
3. Tissue pressure transiently mounts within this confined space, rapidly relaxing to its original state.
4. The entire tip-columellar complex advances relative to the caudal end of the septum posteriorly as the membranous septum contributes to this deprojection-reprojection movement of the tip.

These anatomic considerations suggest similar strategies to (1) optimize postsurgical softness of the tip and to (2) maintain its ability to absorb shock.

The soft tissue sanctuaries are preserved and spared dissection; skeletal grafting of these spaces is avoided to the fullest extent possible. At least 4 mm of membranous septum between the medial crura and the caudal end of the septum is maintained. Rotation and projection are controlled with bilateral anterior septal tunnels, bilateral release of the perispinal attachments, and advancement of the tip-columellar complex relative to the septum. When a long caudal end limits rotation, it is shortened appropriately. Slight overcorrection of tip projection may be required in order to minimize a slight tendency of the tip to deproject postoperatively. Occurrence of a polly beak deformity can be reliably avoided and should not be quoted as a prominent or typical risk of the endonasal operation. In congenital and advanced revisional cases in which the columella is short or there is substantial soft tissue contracture, the technique may require compromise and a shallower columellar pocket may become necessary.

Grafting of the interdomal space is avoided, whenever possible. When recontouring and approximation of the domes is required, variations of Pastorek-type interdomal sutures are placed, with care taken to preserve an adequate proportion of interdomal space and to maintain mobility of the domes relative to each other.

Filleting dissection of the soft triangle down to the alar rim is avoided. When modification is required, this is achieved with an appropriately shaped and placed alar strut graft, which may be positioned with a guiding suture threaded through the alar rim at the level of the soft triangle.

The cartilage-void infracrural (fibromuscular) portion of the alar rim is handled in similar fashion. When transposition of the grafted lateral crus is performed, dissection is limited inferolaterally and an appropriate cuff of soft tissue is preserved.

Third cardinal principle: restructure the lower lateral cartilages– to appear natural
Traditional educational systems usually emphasize straight thinking, as is shown in the observation of early development: toddlers paint round shapes without instruction. Placing letters along a straight line, drawing with a ruler, and calculating the area of angular geometric forms become omnipresent during further schooling but are not natural. One of the great modern contrarians of has shown how organic forms can shape ingenious architecture. Antoni Gaudi's academy director commented on Gaudi's graduation with the words: "Who knows, if we have presented our diploma to an insane or to a genius. Only time will tell."

If Gaudi had been an early pioneer rhinoplasty surgeon, the thinking would be different. Curved structures serve important purposes in nature. Although a linear beam does not give way when subjected to load, a curved structure bends and recoils to its original shape. Gaudi did not incorporate straight beams into his work. The anatomic structures of the preseptal deformation zone (as shown in **Fig. 6**A–D) would likely have fascinated all of Gaudi's senses.

The concept of nasal tip recontouring goes hand in hand with the ECR It allows treatment of the LLC like a malleable metallic band, permitting its reshaping without transection. The ability to form a new domal angle and eliminate undesirable curvatures such as lateral crural convexities or the old domal angle lends surgeons an infinite armamentarium when correcting nasal tip deformities. One essential element of the concept is the preservation of the curved medial crura within their network of soft tissue fibers. Midline dissection of the preseptal deformation zone and placement of linear supporting grafts such as columellar struts is reserved for infrequent scenarios with unusual deficits in projection (eg, cleft deformities). The configuration of the domal angles is controlled with fine scoring and intradomal and interdomal sutures. The shape of the lateral crus is controlled with variations of alar strut grafts, folding techniques, and (frequent) transposition of the lateral crus. Changes in shape, placement, and orientation of the (grafted) lateral crus allow for correction of virtually all deformities of the ala, including alar retraction, valve disorders, and deviations associated with malposition of the lateral crus. Similar to the medial crus, a natural curvature of the lateral crus is preserved by bending the graft-crus construct during placement of the adapting mattress sutures. The resulting shear between the 2 laminae forces the lateral crus into a natural bend to best recreate nature.

Fourth cardinal principle: limit to 4 autologous graft types
A large number of grafting techniques have been reported. It is presumed that most reported techniques can achieve the effect they are designed for. However, for learning surgeons, 2 difficulties arise. First, many techniques require substantial experience and knowledge of minute detail in order to work well. Second, it is almost impossible to learn the best selection of one technique over another. For example, no data have ever convincingly shown which variation of a spreader graft is best indicated under which circumstances.

The limitation to 4 types of grafts has developed without particular intent. Modifications of lateral crural strut grafts in combination with the concept of natural-looking recontouring of the LLCs allows addressing all relevant deformities of the tip-ala complex. This observation has marginalized all other graft types in that anatomic region in my practice. Reconstruction of the septum, spreader grafting, and grafting to modify dorsal height and contour are the other remaining essential grafting techniques in my practice. The avoidance of all nonautologous grafts and implants has eliminated all potential risks associated with these materials.

The concept of using only the 4 grafting techniques described here has important advantages for learning surgeons:

1. The decision-making process is streamlined.
2. Mastery of individual techniques can be achieved earlier, because learning surgeons can focus on a more limited number of techniques. Repetition becomes more frequent and thus it is hoped that the learning curve becomes steeper.
3. Analysis of the effects of grafting techniques is facilitated, because their effects can be associated with a more limited number of maneuvers.

The following 4 essential grafting techniques are foundational to the S.O.F.T. concept.

First graft type: septal stenting and reconstruction grafts One key to successful endonasal rhinoplasty is the reconstruction of the septum within its natural confines and dimensions. In particular, the caudal end is placed where it would be if the nose was in an unaltered state, of naturally beautiful form, and with ideal function.

Important technical principles to achieve these goals include the swinging-door technique for deviations in the sagittal plane and appropriate strip resections along the base and the caudal end. Correction of complex deformities, including twisting and fractures, can be approached in a segmental approach. Release of the upper lateral cartilages often facilitates analysis of the deformity; single targeted incisions are then placed where needed in order to eliminate all relevant memory and to allow the septum to regain its original shape. Weakening of septal cartilage with crushing or scoring techniques is avoided. Segmental stenting techniques with spreader, stenting, and partial replacement grafts are used in order to obtain a straight, thin, and (when possible) complete septum. Appropriately shaped and thinned grafts of cartilage, perpendicular plate, and occasionally auricular cartilage are fixated with Monocryl or polydioxanone (PDS) mattress sutures, typically in side-to-side fashion. When the width of the septum becomes an issue (usually around region 2), end-to-end placements with reinforcing stenting (spreader) grafts may be preferable. Bilaminar opposing conchal cartilage grafts (and PDS plate reconstruction) can allow for reconstruction of advanced disorder.[10] Only when these are insufficient is harvest of costal cartilage pursued. Mastery of adequate exposure through a combined hemitransfixion and intercartilaginous incision; release of the upper lateral cartilages (ULCs); proper selection of spreader and other stenting grafts; preparation of posterior septal, bilaminar conchal cartilage and perpendicular plate grafts; use of costal cartilage grafts; and occasional application of PDS foil are all the elements of the surgical spectrum required to address most septal disorders.

Second graft type: spreader grafts Reconstruction of the middle third has been claimed to prevent disharmony between the bony and the cartilaginous dorsum in reduction rhinoplasty, especially with extended follow-up.

Data by Tasman[11] and the impressive experience by Pastorek[12] may challenge this claim. Excellent long-term results have been reported by reputable surgeons in reduction rhinoplasty without the use of spreader grafts. Spreader grafts are also harvest hungry and carry their own risks and difficulties.

In 2006, I published a systematic, structured depiction of various spreader graft types in the sagittal view.[13] Subsequently, a large number of variations of spreader grafts have been reported. However, reliable data to allow for selection of the appropriate modification of spreader graft reconstruction are lacking and likely impossible to ever generate, given the important variations of tissue-related and surgeon-related factors and the limitations of diagnosing the type of deformity in a standardized fashion. It therefore becomes incumbent on experienced surgeons to choose the appropriate variation of conventional, adapted, folded, or otherwise modified spreader grafts for each case, based on experience and judgment. The following principles can aid in selecting the appropriate spreader graft:

1. In the absence of a wide middle third, spreader graft reconstruction of the middle third is beneficial for the long-term cosmetic outcome.
2. Lateral asymmetries of the middle third should be addressed with spreader graft techniques, rather than by placing augmentation grafts over the ULCs.
3. The conventional spreader graft lends a more defined contour to the middle third, compared with the spreader flap technique.
4. Avoiding spreader grafts after dorsal reduction is possible in selected scenarios, with advanced surgical technique and extensive experience. I place and suture fixate spreader grafts in more than 90% of cases in which the ULCs are released from the septum.
5. Variations of the pushdown/letdown technique represent an alternative to middle third reconstruction. Having been trained by Eugene Kern in these techniques first hand, I have used them throughout my career in a small proportion of reduction rhinoplasties. Their obvious advantage is the preservation of dorsal surface. Disadvantages include wider exposure, more extensive osteotomies with increased bruising and swelling, introduction of instability in previously fixed landmarks, notable deviations from the midline, narrowing of the piriform aperture, and limitations in the ability to modify the inherent contour of the dorsum. Similarly, the Skoog technique can offer important advantages and likely allows the correction of the most dorsal irregularities, as elegantly shown through the endonasal approach by Constantinidis and Fyrmpas.[14] The risk profile seems more benign than that of the pushdown/letdown and includes midline shift and contour irregularities at the transition zones. The spare-roof technique described by Goncalves and colleagues preserves the entire continuity of the ULCs across the midline. Risks include reelevation of the framework and ballooning of the ULCs.[15] In very experienced hands, as with most techniques, the risks of the listed techniques can be well controlled. Thus, the risk/benefit ratio can be shifted so favorably that these techniques can find application in a larger proportion of cases. Given the intent to present a simplified didactic concept, I suggest for the present discussion that:
   a. Dorsal reduction and spreader graft reconstruction of the middle third should remain the first technique to teach learning surgeons, because it is the easiest to learn and conceptualize.
   b. None of the above-listed techniques (spreader grafting, pushdown/letdown, Skoog, spare roof) exceeds the limits of what can be reliably achieved through an endonasal operation.
   c. The roof-sparing techniques likely deserve increased study. Given the currently available body of evidence, none of the above-listed techniques has been shown to be superior. Likely, they are satisfactory methods of controlling dorsal height and will find a balanced representation among dorsal reduction techniques.

Third graft type: laminar lateral crural grafting with addition of the stairstep graft and the foundation graft This graft type is composed of variations and lateral extensions of the lateral crural strut graft.

The ECR approach allows powerful modification of all relevant tip deformities. With recontouring of the lateral crus, repositioning of the domal angle, placement of variations of intradomal and interdomal sutures, reorientation of the lateral crus, and placement of lateral crural strut grafts of varying shape, virtually all deformities of the tip and ala can be reliably addressed. One important advantage of the ECR is efficient reduction of an important risk associated with the delivery approach: after completion of the delivery approach and placement of an interdomal suture, the nasal valve angle may be narrowed by transmission of tension from the domal region to the scroll. Complete release of all tension-banding effects and placement of a lateral crural strut graft through the ECR neutralizes this effect and lends support to the nasal valve. In addition, the risk of accentuation of the alar fold is minimized.

Preliminary retrospective data extracted from the Regensburg Rhinoplasty Database show the importance of this effect: patients who underwent alar strut graft placement through an ECR approach showed significantly improved nasal airway scores compared with the delivery approach. A complete discussion of these data is beyond the scope of the present discussion and is reported in detail in a subsequent article.

Extensions of the alar strut graft to be included in this segment are the stairstep graft, which allows further lateralization of the nasal valve angle in valve repair (**Fig. 7**), and the foundation graft, which allows building a symmetric bony base in cleft repair.[16] In cases in which important substance deficits of the LLC are identified, replacement grafts or facet grafts as described by Tobias[17] are used. The principle of laminar grafting (ie, placement of flat grafts to reconstitute, support, or reconstruct the natural shape and contour of the LLC) is consistently upheld. When feasible, shearing fixation is pursued in order to achieve a natural curvature of the stented lateral crus. Placement of augmentation grafts to protrude from the surface of the LLCs (like shield or cap grafts) is not pursued.

Fourth graft type: dorsal augmentation and camouflage grafts

Camouflage grafts It is important to differentiate between augmentation and camouflage grafts. Camouflage grafts include crushed, scratched, shaved, and diced cartilage as well as various types of fascia, perichondrium, and dermis. Crushing and scratching cartilage destroys extracellular matrix and chondrocytes and introduces varying, unpredictable degrees of resorption as well as a risk of ingrowth into overlying dermis. In contrast, diced or shaved cartilage grafts are both produced by sharp transection, which preserves the integrity of the extracellular matrix and embedded chondrocytes. These grafts are therefore more desirable and more predictable. Diced cartilage is excellent to correct minor irregularities when cut ultrafine, placed under direct vision, and fixated with a small volume of fibrin glue. When the skin is thin, an extra layer of fascia helps to further smoothen contour. Over time, experience has shown that camouflage grafts in general do not reliably fill irregularities of more than 1 mm.

In revisional procedures, skin damage may be present as a result of dermal injury. Signs include telangiectasias and thin, glistening, dyspigmented areas of skin. Such changes are very difficult to improve. The first order of priority is time-consuming, meticulous skin elevation. Among multiple techniques used to treat skin atrophy, free dermal grafting has become my preferred method. With placement as the superficial most grafting layer, dermis has the potential to regenerate atrophic skin changes, likely by replacement of dermis with the same tissue type. This regeneration can be near complete in some cases.

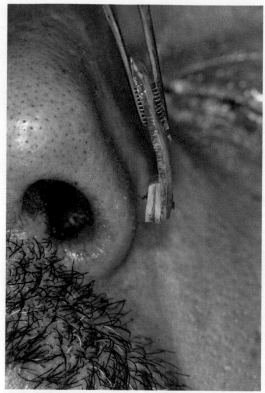

Fig. 7. Lateral crural strut grafts with 2 stairstep grafts. These grafts allow more effective lateralization of the lateral crus and thus allow more pronounced opening of the nasal valve area in nasal valve correction.

Dorsal augmentation grafts For more substantial dorsal defects and saddle nose correction, reconstruction of the dorsal septum and its transition to the upper lateral cartilages is first priority. This treatment usually entails correction and strengthening of the dorsal strut and placement of conventional spreader grafts. If an important deficit in dorsal projection remains, the defect is shaped to provide a straight and even foundation. The dorsum can then be further augmented and contoured with glued dice (Tasman technique) or diced cartilage in fascia (DCIF).[18,19] Problems with sagging, shifting, and deformation of DCIF can be controlled with the following methods: the graft is based on a flat (not concave) foundation and the fascial sleeve is held in place with 4 transcutaneous positioning sutures. It is then filled in situ with fine dice and 1 component of fibrin glue; the second component is injected percutaneously. The graft is then molded and the proximal end closed by tying the purse-string suture; additional fixation is achieved by cementing its flanks with dice and fibrin glue under direct vision. When preexisting skin damage is identified, the surgeon can resort to the DCID (diced cartilage in dermis) graft. For this technique, a dermal sleeve is created and used in the same fashion as described for the DCIF graft. For saddle nose deformities with preexisting atrophic skin damage, this is suggested as an excellent method. **Fig. 8**A–D shows placement of a DCID graft filled with conchal cartilage to revise dorsal irregularities resulting from a previously placed rigid costal cartilage graft.

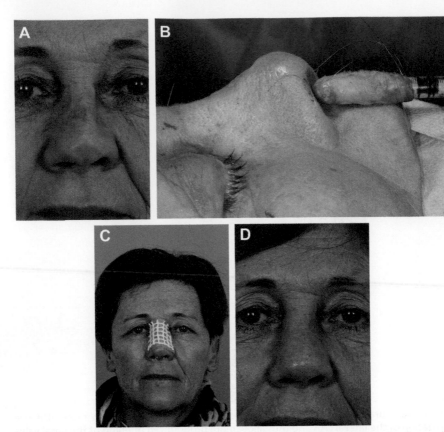

Fig. 8. (*A*) Preoperative appearance of deformed costal cartilage dorsal graft, after multiple previous procedures to repair a severe posttraumatic saddle nose deformity. (*B*) Revisional procedure with placement of a DCID graft filled with diced conchal cartilage. (*C*) The procedure was performed in an ambulatory setting, and the surgery was inconspicuous to the public after 8 days. (*D*) One year postoperative appearance with smooth and symmetric dorsal contour. Skin color and texture had recovered markedly. Revision of the tip was not requested.

Fifth cardinal principle: conserve anatomic structures within their habitats

The S.O.F.T. concept has evolved with ongoing efforts to conserve nasal anatomy. The guiding principle has been to respect and, where needed, recreate the soft tissue compartmentalization and structural framework of the nose as established by nature. In particular, the following structures are conserved to the greatest extent possible:

- The septal cartilage as foreseen by nature
- The septal space
- The columellar and lateral nasal neurovascular bundles
- The anatomic continuity of the LLCs
- The membranous septum and preseptal deformation zone

Emphasis is placed on respecting the habitats of cartilaginous entities within the confines foreseen by nature. These entities include the septal space, the interdomal space, the soft triangles, and the fibromuscular tissues of the alae. Grafts that extend anteriorly into the membranous septum, such as columellar strut and septal extension grafts, grafts that extend into the interdomal space, such as shield and cap grafts, and grafts that extend into the facets or the fibromuscular tissues of the alae, such as rim grafts, are avoided and replaced with the alternative techniques described earlier. Corrections in the dimensions of the septal cartilage to include basal, posterior, and caudal strip resections form part of the concept. These corrections should be fashioned with the goal of creating septal dimensions as nature would have foreseen in a given nose with ideal dimensions and airway.

Sixth cardinal principle: preserve all turbinate soft tissue

A deep respect for the function of the nasal mucosa has been emphasized by Eugene Kern, a leading nasal physiologist and rhinologist. My exclusive technique to reduce turbinate volume has become the selective submucous resection (SMR) of turbinate bone. This method has multiple advantages: medialization of the head of the inferior turbinate with lateral osteotomy can no longer occur and preservation of the Guyuron triangle becomes unnecessary. Thus, curved osteotomies are not required and the more controlled and less traumatic straight osteotomies can be pursued in all cases. Injury to the turbinate mucosa and, more importantly, submucosa is avoided and the full warming and humidifying capacity of the nasal mucosa is preserved. With meticulous suturing, the need for packing is avoided. In a study including 122 patients who underwent rhinoplasty with concomitant turbinate surgery, 121 of the 122 were treated with excellent functional outcome with full preservation of all turbinate soft tissue. One of the 122 required revision surgery with laser treatment of marked submucosal hypertrophy.[20] Therefore, SMR is recommended as the preferred method of turbinate treatment in Caucasian rhinoplasty.

Seventh cardinal principle: apply minimally invasive techniques

Atraumatic technique The Caucasian nose and face scars well, but not ideally. Although the resolution of edema is likely not substantially different among skin types, residual edema and bruising are visible for a longer time in fair and thin Caucasian skin. The following 12 precautionary measures are therefore taken to enhance gentle handling of the soft tissue envelope during the procedure:

1. Preservation of the columellar neurovascular bundle maintains the most important dependent venous and lymphatic drainage pathway of the nose.
2. Well-administered controlled hypotension by an experienced anesthesiologist limits edema very effectively. Systolic blood pressure is held at 90 mm Hg, unless other morbidity poses a contraindication.
3. Use of local anesthesia with sedation, when feasible, enhances early postoperative recovery and seems to further reduce postoperative swelling and bruising.
4. Local anesthesia with adrenaline is injected repeatedly throughout the procedure to minimize stimulation and perfusion. Placement includes the luminal surface of the osteotomy tracts and a circular block around the nose.
5. The skin and face are kept cool with gauze soaked in sterile ice water throughout the procedure.
6. Soft tissue trauma is further reduced by the choice of the most minimally invasive approach, technique, exposure, and instrumentation.
7. The sequence of the procedure is planned so maneuvers associated with more trauma (osteotomies) are performed as late as possible.
8. All wound surfaces are kept moist, and approximation of opposing wound surfaces is maximized during the procedure, thus effectively limiting desiccation injury.

9. Exposure for lateral osteotomies is kept minimal. The use of the Piezo instrument is limited to reduction paramedian osteotomies, fine adjustment of dorsal irregularities, and the management of congenital lateral bony deformities.
10. Only straight osteotomies are performed: paramedian, intermediate, lateral, and transverse percutaneous osteotomies are performed without curve and without fade. This method reliably avoids uncontrolled shatter of bone and minimizes trauma.
11. Meticulous facial plastic surgical technique and the gentlest handling of the tissues are self-evident requirements.
12. Endonasal packing is avoided, thus reducing oncotic pressure and facilitating lymphatic drainage in the early postoperative phase. Tamponade-free surgery is achieved by meticulous hemostasis and complete closure of all endonasal incisions.

Minimal graft harvest Local and distant graft harvest has seen an important expansion over the past 2 decades. The L-strut concept is claimed to justify harvest of a large proportion of the nasal septum. The author analyzed a series of revision rhinoplasties and found data suggesting that harvest of septal cartilage warrants careful consideration.

Using the Regensburg Rhinoplasty Database, 500 consecutive endonasal revisions that underwent primary surgery by another surgeon (not my own revisions) were analyzed (from 01/2013 to 03/2019). With the use of operative drawings and intraoperative notes, the author has consistently (since 2009) documented his subjective perception of the single factor most contributing to the global difficulty of revision procedures. Of note, this coincides with neither the patient's reason to seek revision nor with the most frequent anatomic deformity identified. The top 5 contributing factors were, in order of frequency:

1. Septal cartilage depletion (184 out of 500)
2. Compromised/scarred/missing endonasal lining tissue (86 out of 500)
3. Compromised/scarred external skin–soft tissue envelope (78 out of 500)
4. Transection or significant compromise of the LLCs (63 out of 500)
5. Compromise/lack of reconstruction of the middle third (57 out of 500)

The harvest of costal cartilage carries risk and morbidity, albeit these are acceptable in experienced hands. Moreover, costal cartilage has profoundly different tissue characteristic than septal cartilage: it is firmer, subject to warping, and can contribute to increased postsurgical stiffness of the nasal tip.

With depletion of septal cartilage being the most important factor making revision surgery difficult, and costal cartilage being a material not ideally suited for nasal physiology, emphasis has been placed on developing strategies to minimize the use of septal and costal cartilage, both in primary and in revisional cases. These strategies include:

1. More liberal use of conchal cartilage and other tissues (temporalis fascia), especially for volume and camouflage grafting.
2. Use of bilaminar opposing conchal cartilage grafts for caudal septal reconstruction.
3. Reduction in the height of spreader grafts used.
4. More liberal use of perpendicular plate grafting.
5. Use of PDS plate septal reconstruction.

It is emphasized that the thoughtful use of both septal and costal cartilage remains well justified. With more attention placed on the techniques listed earlier, the need for costal cartilage grafting in revisional cases has been reduced in my own practice by about 50% (from 60–70 annually to 20–30 annually).

With very infrequent exceptions, I routinely preserve at least two-thirds of the residual septal cartilage in my own primary procedures. When more cartilage is required, I resort to other sources. Scoring, crushing, or other injury to residual cartilage is strictly avoided.

In this context, a critical note regarding the L-strut concept is in order: this concept lends justification to learning surgeons harvesting most of the septal cartilage for grafting. Instead of the L-strut concept, a concept of maximal septal preservation with application of the methods listed earlier is suggested.

When necessary, septal reconstruction is performed to the minimal extent required. Partial in situ reconstruction has been shown to be consistently sufficient. Placement of stenting grafts, perpendicular plate grafts, bilaminar conchal grafts, and (when inevitable) costal cartilage grafts allows reliable anatomic reconstruction. Those revision procedures in which most of the septal cartilage has been preserved without injury are among the easiest and least extensive procedures in my practice. Thus, septal conservation is stressed as an important principle in rhinoplasty surgery.

Measures to provide quick and comfortable recovery The following factors have been identified to enhance patient satisfaction and shorten postoperative recovery:

- Avoidance of nasal packing, with the ideal goal of providing a patent nasal airway as early as the first night after surgery
- Early removal of septal splints on day 2 or 3 after surgery
- Early removal of the nasal cast, usually 1 week after surgery
- Preference of an ambulatory setting
- Preferred use of local anesthesia with sedation, when feasible

Illustrative case studies

The following cases highlight the tremendous variability and potency of the ECR approach, paired with the concept of nasal tip recontouring in Caucasian rhinoplasty.

Fig. 9 shows a patient who underwent the ECR approach with recontouring of the LLCs, repositioning of maloriented LLCs, recontouring of the domal angles, and placement of alar strut grafts, with 3-year follow-up. The patient's airway was ideal, and her request of preserving a naturally appearing, nonoperated look was met. Of note, anatomic types closely related to the Caucasian nose, such as this patient, can also be managed according to the principles presented here.

Fig. 10 shows a 19-year-old male patient with a unilateral cleft lip deformity. This patient underwent an endonasal approach, partial septal replacement, and foundation graft placement with costal cartilage transfer and staged revision cheiloplasty. The 3-year follow-up results show the powerful tools endonasal rhinoplasty can provide in complex congenital and revisional scenarios.

DISCUSSION

The S.O.F.T. concept detailed in this article applies to Caucasian and closely related anatomy only. Other ethnic types, such as the thicker skin of the African and Asian noses, call for more pronounced structural support and may exceed what the endonasal S.O.F.T. concept can achieve in the Caucasian type of nose.

The present article departs in some aspects from established teachings. However, this should not be interpreted as a criticism of the open or other endonasal concepts. It is emphasized that the operation (endonasal or open) entails the most profound diverging effects on the dynamic interaction between skeleton and the skin–soft tissue

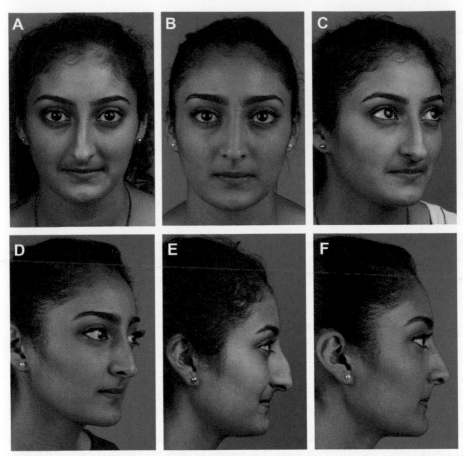

Fig. 9. Representative case of correction of lateral crural malposition, tip ptosis, columellar bifidity, and pronounced tip width. (*A, C, E*) Preoperative views; (*B, D, F*) 3-year postoperative outcome after correction through an ECR approach, re-orientation of malpositioned lateral crura, placement of lateral crural strut grafts, and tip modification through recontouring of the lateral crura with intradomal and interdomal sutures.

envelope. As a result, nature and effects of framework modification follow substantially different rules. Rather than discussing 2 different approaches to the same surgical problem, surgeons should recognize that the endonasal and the open procedures represent 2 entirely different operations. Therefore, diverging methodology should be expected and discussed in a holistic context. The present article molds the Caucasian endonasal operation into an autonomous concept, which should stand alone.

Many concepts in rhinoplasty have been passed on as accepted dogma. Proving or disproving their validity is restricted by important limitations of scientific study in rhinoplasty, because many confounding variables are impossible to control. Alternative concepts have largely replaced the following principles and methods in my practice:

- The L-strut concept
- The columellar strut
- The tongue-in-groove technique
- Tip contour grafting

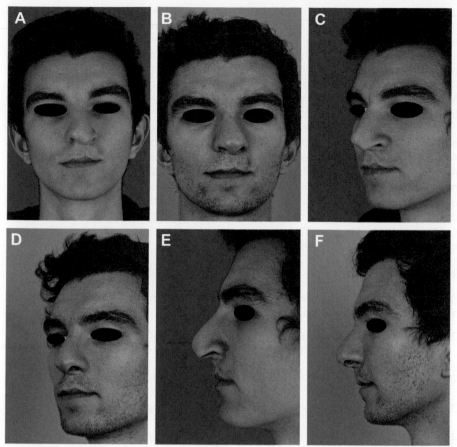

Fig. 10. Representative case of correction of adult unilateral cleft nasal deformity. (*A, C, E*) Preoperative views; (*B, D, F*) 3-year postoperative outcome after ECR approach, costal cartilage transfer, placement of unilateral left foundation graft, bilateral alar strut grafts, recontouring of the lateral crura, and revision cheiloplasty.

- The lateral Piezo osteotomy
- Submucous turbinate reduction
- Cartilage crushing and aggressive scoring
- Suture-based techniques of valve correction

My own level V experience cannot justify claiming that the alternatives presented are superior. However, an open-minded, critical reconsideration of these techniques is suggested.

Valve surgery is one of the many examples in which clinicians have not substantially overcome the limits of level V evidence. Friedman and colleagues[21] provide an excellent review of many established techniques. However, most investigators rely on 1 or 2 favorite techniques, based on their own positive experience. The stairstep graft, combined with an alar strut graft of sufficient structure, has become my personal workhorse and has marginalized all other methods of valve repair in my practice.

Teaching and training endonasal rhinoplasty has witnessed a substantial decline over the past 2 decades. Constantian and Martin's[22] observations are excellent and a recommended read. One important reason is the perceived greater difficulty to learn the procedure. It is my hope that the concepts summarized under the fourth cardinal principle can help surgeons to better understand and learn endonasal rhinoplasty. Many of the surgeons who have visited me in Regensburg have given encouraging feedback as they have integrated endonasal concepts into their practice. Mastering the ECR approach is key to unlocking many complex deformities with little effort. Most surgeons experienced with open rhinoplasty report being comfortable with the ECR after a handful of procedures.

The data presented earlier show the outcome of the same surgeon obtained from intervals when (almost) 100% open versus endonasal operations were performed. All of the important confounding variables remained stable over the study period. Although outcome data in rhinoplasty will never equal the quality other disciplines can generate, there is every reason to conclude that the endonasal operation obtains equivalent outcomes. Whether it is justified to address the most complex revisional cases endonasally may be controversial. However, this operation should be strongly considered for addressing simple primary scenarios, given its great potential for atraumatic, minimally invasive, and conservative surgery.

SUMMARY

It is my hope that the experiences reported and the data shown justify the following statements for Caucasian rhinoplasty:

1. The endonasal operation achieves equivalent results, both cosmetically and functionally, across the entire spectrum of deformities in the Caucasian type of anatomy.
2. A conservative, atraumatic, and sparing approach with regard to graft harvest and placement is feasible.
3. The goal of achieving a soft feel to the operated nose can be integrated into a treatment concept.
4. Recreation of the skeletal framework as foreseen by nature can serve as an important guiding principle in rhinoplasty.
5. A lean and coherent didactic concept can be presented to learning surgeons, which should facilitate integration of the endonasal operation into any rhinoplasty practice.
6. Turbinate soft tissue can be spared entirely.
7. Ambulatory setting, tamponade-free surgery, and abbreviated recovery are realistic goals.
8. Endonasal and open should not be regarded as different approaches to the same procedure but as entirely separate operations.

DISCLOSURE

Funding for the art work was provided "Facial Plastic Surgery Europe e.V."

REFERENCES

1. Johnson CM, Toriumi DM. Open structure rhinoplasty. Ann Arbor (MI): Saunders; 1990.
2. Toriumi DM. Structure rhinoplasty: lessons learned in 30 years. Chicago: DMT Solutions; 2019.
3. Moore EJ, Kern EB. Atrophic rhinitis: a review of 242 cases. Am J Rhinol 2001; 15(6):355–61.

4. Sherris DA, Murakami CS. Five things oculoplastic surgeons should know about facial plastic surgery. Ophthalmic Plast Reconstr Surg 1999;15(4):229–31.
5. Gubisch W. The extracorporeal septum plasty: a technique to correct difficult nasal deformities. Plast Reconstr Surg 1995;95(4):672–82.
6. Gubisch W. Twenty-five years experience with extracorporeal septoplasty. Facial Plast Surg 2006;22(4):230–9.
7. Fuleihan NS. The transvestibular approach: a new horizon in rhinoplasty. Arch Facial Plast Surg 2006;8(4):273–82.
8. Gassner HG, Mueller-Vogt U, Strutz J, et al. Nasal tip recontouring in primary rhinoplasty: the endonasal complete release approach. JAMA Facial Plast Surg 2013;15(1):11–6.
9. Available at: www.facial-plastic-surgery.eu. November 1, 2019.
10. Haack S, Gubisch W. Reconstruction of the septum with an autogenous double-layered conchal L-strut. Aesthetic Plast Surg 2014;38(5):912–22.
11. Tasman AJ. Endonasal techniques in revision rhinoplasty. Presented at "Advances in Rhinoplasty", AAFPRS, Orlando, FL, April 5, 2019.
12. Pastorek N, Ham J. The underprojecting nasal tip: an endonasal approach. Facial Plast Surg Clin North Am 2004;12(1):93–106.
13. Gassner HG, Friedman O, Sherris DA, et al. An alternative method of middle vault reconstruction. Arch Facial Plast Surg 2006;8(6):432–5.
14. Constantinidis J, Fyrmpas G. Reinserting the hump in primary rhinoplasty: the gain is three-fold. Plast Reconstr Surg Glob Open 2016;4(10):e1021.
15. Ferreira MG, Monteiro D, Reis C, et al. Spare roof technique: a middle third new technique. Facial Plast Surg 2016;32(01):111–6.
16. Gassner HG, Schwan F, Haubner F, et al. Technique in cleft rhinoplasty: the foundation graft. Facial Plast Surg 2016;32(2):213–8.
17. Tobias GW. Modified universal tiplasty: closed structure rhinoplasty as it pertains to the overprojected and the broad tip. Facial Plast Surg 1994;10(4):389–98.
18. Tasman AJ. Replacement of the nasal dorsum with a diced cartilage glue graft. Facial Plast Surg 2019;35(1):53–7.
19. Daniel RK, Calvert JW. Diced cartilage grafts in rhinoplasty surgery. Plast Reconstr Surg 2004;113(7):2156–71.
20. Rudes M, Schwan F, Klass F, et al. Turbinate reduction with complete preservation of mucosa and submucosa during rhinoplasty. HNO 2018;66(2):111–7.
21. Friedman O, Cekic E, Gunel C. Functional rhinoplasty. Facial Plast Surg Clin North Am 2017;25(2):195–9.
22. Constantian MB, Martin JP. Why can't more good surgeons learn rhinoplasty? Aesthet Surg J 2015;35(4):486–9.

Open Structure Approach to the European or Caucasian Nose

David A. Sherris, MD

KEYWORDS

- Rhinoplasty • Open rhinoplasty • Caucasian nose • Nasal valve
- Thin-skin rhinoplasty • Tension nose deformity • Hanging columella • Crooked nose

KEY POINTS

- Open structure rhinoplasty is a technique of rhinoplasty that through the external approach uses grafts and sutures to obtain a structurally and functionally sound result.
- The tripod concept of nasal tip dynamics and understanding tip support mechanisms are the keys to this approach.
- Thin skin provides a dilemma to the rhinoplasty surgeon that must be overcome.
- The overprojected nose, tension nose, dorsal hump, and excess columellar show will be faced by every surgeon and can all be treated effectively.
- Nasal valve anatomy and abnormalities must be understood to perform successful rhinoplasty in any patient.

 Video content accompanies this article at http://www.oto.theclinics.com.

The term European or Caucasian nose is an area of debate in the literature for nomenclature regarding medical research.[1] However, because this is an article on rhinoplasty, not cardiac disease or other systemic disorders, please accept the limitations of the terminology. The author uses these terms in this publication for simplification purposes.

Open structure rhinoplasty is a term popularized by Calvin Johnson Jr, MD and Dean Toriumi, MD in their book published in 1990.[2] The philosophy of open structure rhinoplasty is to restore or maintain structural support of the cartilaginous and bony nasal skeleton while altering the shape to improve aesthetics of the nose.[3] Function is also improved or preserved when applying the techniques to achieve the aesthetic goals.

The lower third of the nose is approached by applying the tripod concept.[2–4] The combined medial crus and each lateral crus, along with their ligamentous and fibrous

Department of Otolaryngology, Jacobs School of Medicine and Biomedical Sciences, 1237 Delaware Avenue, Buffalo, NY 14209, USA
E-mail address: dsherris@buffalo.edu

Otolaryngol Clin N Am 53 (2020) 237–254
https://doi.org/10.1016/j.otc.2019.12.003
0030-6665/20/Published by Elsevier Inc.

oto.theclinics.com

attachments, each represent 1 leg of the tripod. By altering the tripod appropriately, the nose can be deprojected, projected, rotated, or derotated. As the surgeon operates on the tip, he or she must also be aware of the major and minor tip supports.[5,6] Important tip supports include the caudal and dorsal septum, the lower lateral cartilages (LLCs), the scroll between the upper lateral cartilage (ULC) and the LLCs, the interdomal ligaments, the membranous septum, the sesamoid cartilages and their fibrous attachment to the pyriform aperture, the skin soft tissue attachments to the cartilage, the caudal end of the ULC, and the nasal spine. The importance of each tip support structure varies depending on the anatomic abnormalities and variations one faces in examining each nose.[7] However, surgeons must keep in mind that many rhinoplasty maneuvers, starting with separating the skin and soft tissue envelope from the underlying structures, and including but not limited to cephalic trim, dome division, separating the interdomal ligament, disrupting the membranous septum, and such all weaken tip support. Open structure rhinoplasty is based on rebuilding the structural support during the surgery with suture and grafting techniques aimed at restoring the structural integrity and improving the aesthetics. Common techniques to achieve these goals include placing septal/columellar sutures, columellar struts, tip grafts, alar batten grafts, tip sutures, septal spreader grafts, or using the tongue-and-groove technique to support the tip on the caudal septum.[2–4,6–10] These techniques and others are discussed in this article in relation to specific dilemmas the surgeon faces more commonly in the European or Caucasian nose.

Issues the surgeon faces more frequently in the European or Caucasian nose than in other ethnic or racial group noses include but are not limited to the following:

- Thin skin
- Overprojected tip
- Hanging columella
- Dorsal hump
- Tension nose
- Nasal valve obstruction
- Crooked nose

This article addresses common techniques to many of these issues in a case-based evaluation. By no means does this article attempt to provide the only answers to these common dilemmas. Rather, the techniques presented represent those that have served this author well over 25 years in practice.

THIN SKIN

Early in a rhinoplasty surgeon's career, one discovers the difficulties associated with the thin-skinned nose in rhinoplasty. Every existing irregularity is visible and typically bothers the patient. Likewise, any alteration to the existing underlying cartilaginous and bony structure of the nose has the potential to provide new opportunities for visible irregularities postoperatively. Dorsal irregularity at the bone cartilage junction, visible tip graft, and difficulty in camouflaging minor asymmetries are amplified in this patient population. Some valid options to deal with this specific problem include trying to thicken the skin with various dorsal implants, avoiding rigid grafts, and avoiding significant dorsal manipulations to minimize the risk.

Skin thickening agents that have stood the test of time include fascia grafts (temporalis, fascia lata), perichondrial grafts (especially when harvesting rib), and allografts (acellular human dermal matrix)[8,11] (**Figs. 1** and **2**). The difficulty with autografts is that they require a secondary harvest site remote from the primary surgical site, resulting in increased operative time, costs, and secondary morbidity. However, these

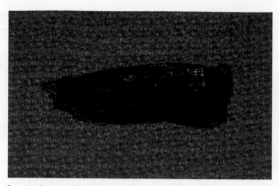

Fig. 1. Temporalis fascia, layered and partially dried for dorsal camouflage.

grafts are the most reliable because they are harvested from the patient, and their take level is unequaled.

The advantage of allografts is that they come off of the shelf and do not add time or secondary morbidity to the case. However, they can face a slightly higher rate of resorption than autograft and thus provide less reliable long-term outcomes.[11] Certainly allograft should not be depended on for major augmentation or structural graft use. However, to camouflage dorsal irregularities, they are very useful.

Tip grafts and other rigid grafts can be used in thin-skinned patients if necessary. Patients in which tip plication sutures cause nasal valve obstruction by pushing the LLC into the nasal cavity represent such a case (**Fig. 3**A). Dome division, resection of a few millimeters of interdomal cartilage, and suture reconstitution narrows the bulbous tip and preserves the nasal valve area. (**Fig. 3**B). Many surgeons who do dome division then place a tip graft to restabilize the nasal tip (**Fig. 4**A). In these cases, the surgeon must make sure to bevel the edges and even consider morselizing the graft to make it softer. These maneuvers make the graft less likely to become visible over time. The morselized cap graft can be used in thin-skinned patients to provide better tip protection and definition while minimizing the risk of the appearance of a tombstone of a shield graft.[3] In addition, fascia or acellular human dermal matrix graft can be draped over the tip graft to thicken the skin and better camouflage the graft[11] (**Fig. 4**B). If skin-thickening agents are draped over the tip, they should be suture fixated to the cartilage with 6-0 absorbable sutures to prevent migration or contraction

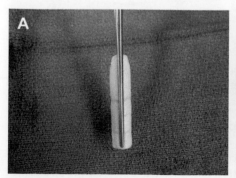
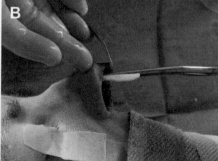

Fig. 2. (*A*) Acellular human dermal matrix cut and rehydrated for placement on the nasal dorsum. (*B*) Allograft being placed through the external approach.

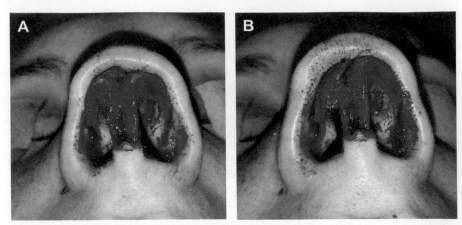

Fig. 3. (*A*) Plication suture of the right nasal tip is causing the lateral aspect of the LLC to obstruct the airway. (*B*) Dome division, resection of a few millimeters of the right dome cartilage, and suture reconstitution narrows the tip while maintaining nasal airway patency.

during healing. Those grafts placed on the dorsum are in a tight pocket and do not usually require suture fixation.

OVERPROJECTED NASAL TIP

The overprojected nasal tip is a common issue in the European or Caucasian nose. Other ethnic groups tend to have the opposite dilemma, with underprojected nasal tip and commonly low nasal dorsum. Tip overprojection can be an isolated dilemma or it can be associated with a tension nose.

Isolated tip overprojection can be treated with a variety of techniques, including freeing the medial crural feet completely from the caudal septum and letting them settle downward.[9] Another common option is to do a dome division, resection, or

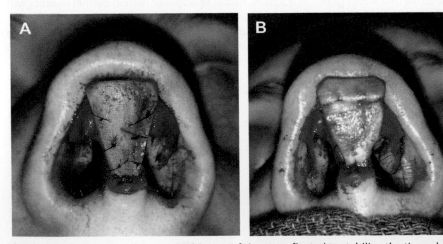

Fig. 4. (*A*) After dome division, a shield tip graft is suture fixated to stabilize the tip and provide an aesthetically pleasing projection. (*B*) If a skin-thickening agent is draped over the tip, it should be suture fixated to prevent contracture.

overlay, and suture reconstitution to preserve tip support. Dome division and resection refers to cutting and removal of a portion of the LLCs at the junction of the medial and lateral crus. Dome division with resection directly at the dome results in deprojection, whereas dome division with resection more lateral to the dome results in tip rotation as well. Finally, dome division with resection more on the medial crus results in derotation and deprojection. These observations are referred to as the tripod concept of nasal tip dynamics.[2–4] Suture reconstitution of the nasal tip after dome division helps to maintain the structural integrity and tip support so that the nose is left with more structural support after surgery than before surgery. A well-supported, structurally sound nose tends to provide an excellent long-term outcome both aesthetically and functionally.

When dome division and suture reconstitution are done, some surgeons advocate overlapping the segments rather than removing them in order to better preserve tip support and structural integrity. Other investigators advocate tip grafting with either shield or cap grafts to both partially reproject the nose in an aesthetically pleasing position and to maintain or improve overall tip strength.[2,3]

HANGING COLUMELLA, DORSAL HUMP, AND TENSION NOSE DEFORMITY

The isolated hanging columella is an uncommon disorder of the nose. One to 2 mm of columellar show below the alar rim is accepted in most cultures as the norm. If a patient presents with excessive columellar show, it is important to evaluate the entire nose for associated problems that may need to be treated (**Fig. 5**).

In cases wherein there is not an enormous amount of excess columellar show, the medial crural feet can be set back on the caudal septum in a tongue-and-groove fashion.[9] The medial crural feet are separated from each other and set back over the caudal septum where they are sutured. This maneuver improves tip support, helps

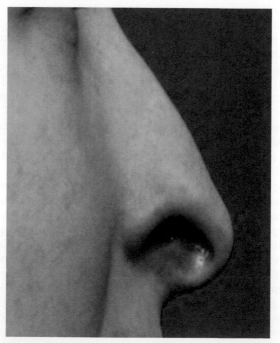

Fig. 5. A patient with severe excess columellar show.

set the tip height, controls tip rotation, and diminishes columellar show. In cases with a greater amount of columellar show, some caudal septal cartilage and mucosa can be resected alone, or in combination with, the tongue-and-groove technique (**Fig. 6**). Both techniques can be used in both the tension nose deformity and the isolated hanging columella technique.

The tension nose deformity is common in both European and Caucasian noses and in the Middle Eastern population. The deformity results from an excessive quadrangular cartilage that causes a large dorsal bump, thin middle third of the nose, excess columella show, and sometimes a ptotic nasal tip.[12] Many times the patient notes that their nasal tip pulls down on smiling. The open septorhinoplasty approach is excellent to treat this deformity because the ULC can be separated on either side of the quadrangular cartilage, allowing resection of the excess dorsal and caudal septum along with excess nasal spine. The depressor septi muscle can also be cut to diminish tip ptosis on smiling. After these maneuvers, the nose relaxes downward toward the face and the nostrils relax from slitlike to a more natural, oval shape. The open approach allows the surgeon to preserve the ULC for use as turn-in spreader flaps if necessary[13] (**Fig. 7A–H**).

The dorsal hump either in the tension nose or in isolated cases is typically resected either piecemeal or in 1 piece. By appropriately projecting the tip initially in an underprojected nose, many times the amount of bump resection needed is lessened.[2,3] Dorsal humps can be large, small, deviated, straight, wide, or narrow.[14] Correct diagnosis of the bump is necessary for appropriate treatment. Small bumps can usually be addressed with simple rasping. Large bumps may require resection with a Rubin osteotome and rasping. If an open roof ensues from resecting a large bump, it must be addressed to avoid inverted V deformity (**Fig. 8**). In addition, when a large bump is removed, the resulting dorsum is automatically wider. To avoid permanent deformity with the inverted V deformity, osteotomies should be performed in these cases (**Fig. 9**).[15] In the case of a straight dorsum with a small open roof, lateral osteotomies that are complete may well suffice. When a large amount of bone and septal cartilage has to be removed, the osteotomies may need to be combined with spreader flaps or grafts to avoid the inverted V deformity from the middle vault collapse (**Figs. 10** and **11A–F**).[13,16]

In cases with a crooked dorsal bump, the addition of an intermediate osteotomy may be an option (see **Fig. 9**). The intermediate osteotomy is planned on the longer, flatter side of a crooked nose to help align the bones more centrally. Intermediate osteotomies can be placed bilaterally in very wide noses as well. This maneuver also evens the height of the nasal bones. Medial osteotomies can be used in cases of very wide dorsums to maximally narrow the dorsum and mobilize it.

Occasionally, an outfracturing medial osteotomy can be used on the longer, flatter side of the crooked nose to further improve symmetry of the dorsum (**Fig. 9**). This technique can be combined with a thicker spreader graft on the longer, flatter side to improve symmetry.[13–16] When assessing a bump for removal, computer imaging is especially useful for both the patient and the surgeon. Imaging provides the surgeon opportunities to point out asymmetries of the nose and face. Sometimes facial asymmetries make it impossible to make a perfectly straight nose. Pointing this out ahead of time helps the patient to understand the shortcomings of a potential surgery. Imaging a straight dorsum in the profile view versus one with a supratip depression also helps in determining what the patient prefers. The author's patient population tends to prefer a relatively straight dorsum. However, surgeons with other patient populations may find theirs prefer a scooped dorsum. Computer imaging is essential to communicate these nuances and lead to both a happy patient and surgeon.

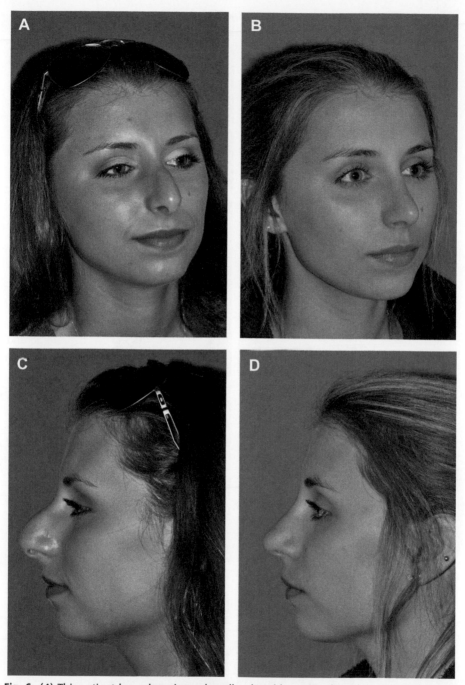

Fig. 6. (*A*) This patient has a hanging columella, dorsal bump, and tension nose without tip ptosis. (*B*) The patient appears 1.5 years after septorhinoplasty. At surgery, 4 mm of caudal septal mucosa and cartilage were resected and the medial crural feet were setback 3 mm. In addition, the patient underwent nasal spine resection, dorsal bump resection, spreader flaps, complete lateral osteotomies, cephalic trim of the LLCs, shield tip graft, and acellular human dermal matrix dorsal overlay. (*C*) Lateral view preoperatively. (*D*) Lateral view 1.5 years later.

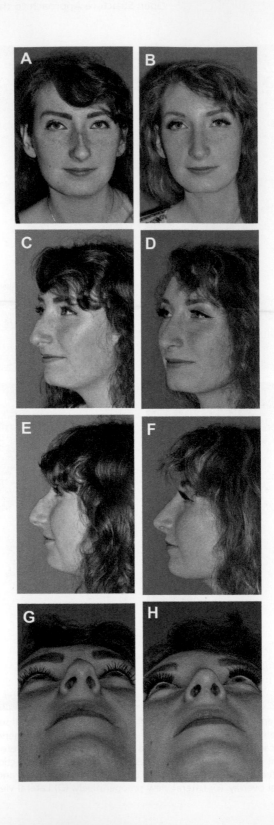

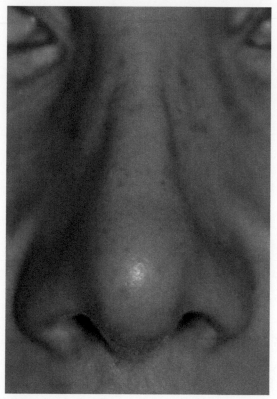

Fig. 8. An open roof and inverted V deformity characterized by thin skin, a visible gap between the upper lateral cartilages, and visible midline dorsal septum.

Recently, some surgeons have reintroduced the push-down technique to improve dorsal humps.[17] The reader is referred to outside sources to further evaluate this technique clearly.

NASAL VALVE OBSTRUCTION

Nasal valve obstruction is a complex collection of many various abnormalities that can be presented either as isolated or in combination. This disorder is the most common cause of nasal obstruction after septoplasty, septorhinoplasty, or rhinoplasty.[18–20] The

◀───

Fig. 7. (*A*) This patient presented with tension nose deformity, thin skin, and a tip that pulled down on smiling pictured in the frontal view. (*B*) The patient appears 1 year after surgery wherein the author performed dorsal hump resection, spreader flaps, dorsal septal resection, nasal spine resection, cutting of the depressor septi muscle, tongue-and-groove setback of the medial crural feet, left alar batten graft, cephalic trim, suture plication of the nasal tip, complete lateral osteotomies, septoplasty, and overlay of the dorsum with acellular human dermal matrix. (*C*) Before surgery in the three-quarter view. (*D*) After surgery in the three-quarter view. (*E*) Before surgery in the profile view. (*F*) After surgery in the profile view. (*G*) Before surgery in the base view. (*H*) After surgery in the base view; note improved shape and symmetry of the nostrils.

Osteotomies

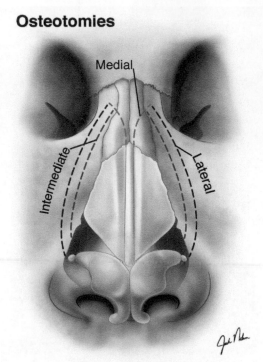

Fig. 9. The typical osteotomies used in rhinoplasty.

problem is more prevalent in the European and Caucasian nose than in other ethnic groups. Because of the multitude of causes and treatments, the reader is referred to rhinoplasty textbooks or many other publications on the subject for a more complete discussion of the subject.

Spreader Flap
A

Spreader Graft
B

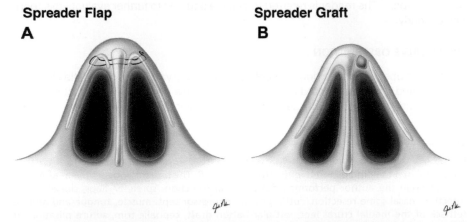

Fig. 10. (*A*) Spreader flaps are residual upper lateral cartilages (ULCs) that are preserved before bump resection. The mucosa off the undersurface is freed with sharp dissection so that they can be turned in and sutured to the lowered, dorsal septum. (*B*) A spreader graft is a rectangular cartilage graft sutured between the ULC and dorsal septum to stabilize the dorsum and open the nasal valve angle.

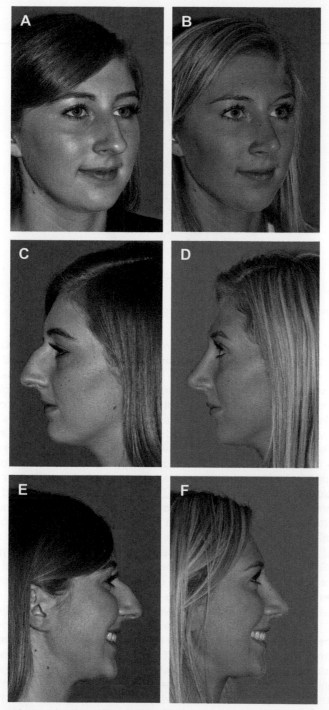

Fig. 11. (*A*) A patient with a large dorsal bump and an overprojected and wide nasal tip. (*B*) One year after septorhinoplasty with dorsal bump resection, spreader flaps, bilateral underlay alar batten grafts, tip suture plication and stabilization sutures, conservative cephalic trim, complete lateral osteotomies, and acellular human dermal matrix graft onlay, the patient is improved aesthetically and functionally. (*C*) Lateral view before surgery. (*D*) Lateral view after surgery. (*E*) Smiling lateral causes tip ptosis. (*F*) After surgery, the tip no longer pulls down on smiling.

Nasal Valve Area

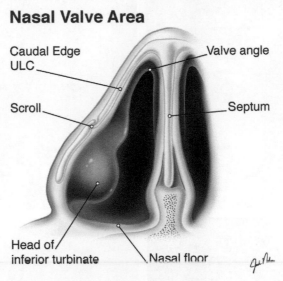

Caudal Edge ULC

Valve angle

Scroll

Septum

Head of inferior turbinate

Nasal floor

Fig. 12. The nasal valve area and its anatomic boundaries.

Succinctly, the valve area refers to the area of highest resistance in the nasal airway (**Fig. 12**). Its borders are the caudal septum, the angle between the ULC and caudal septum, the nasal sidewall, the tip of the inferior turbinate, and the nasal floor.[18,19] Static nasal valve collapse refers to obstruction at rest. Dynamic valve collapse refers to valve obstruction that occurs upon nasal inspiration. Both disorders can be present either as isolated or in combination. When assessing a patient for nasal valve collapse, it is imperative to evaluate the patient both at rest and on forced nasal inspiration. If dynamic collapse is observed, the cotton swab test is useful to assess the contribution of the issue to the overall nasal obstruction symptoms. Using the wooden end of a cotton-tip applicator, the alar cartilages are supported laterally within the nostril while the patient does a forced nasal inspiration (Video 1). If the airway is noted to be especially improved with this maneuver, then dynamic valve collapse is certainly a major contributor to the nasal obstruction. If that is the case, the patient may be instructed to do a nasal strip test at home. The patient is instructed to use a nasal strip both in daytime and at bedtime to see if the airway is improved. Surgery for dynamic valve collapse typically equates the improvement of breathing with the nasal strip. Many times patients will demonstrate a positive Cottle sign, whereby they describe pulling the cheek outward laterally to improve the airway on that side.

The 2 most common causes of nasal valve collapse the author encounters in the European and Caucasian nose are the caudal septal deformity and dynamic alar collapse. The caudal septal deformity can be either congenital or acquired. Because the caudal and dorsal septum are required to preserve nasal support, this problem is difficult to address with standard septoplasty techniques. Rather, caudal septal transplantation and reconstruction are usually required.[21–23] Ideally, septal cartilage is used to reconstitute the caudal septum in a primary case.[21] In severe cases or those in secondary rhinoplasty, alternative materials like rib cartilage, perpendicular plate of the ethmoid and vomer bone, or polydioxanon (PDS) plate with cartilage remnants sewn to it can suffice.[19–23] The open approach provides an easy access to approach the caudal end and suture fixate replacement graft to the ULC, cephalic dorsal strut that is left intact beyond the valve angle, and the nasal spine (**Fig. 13**A–D).[21,24] This

3-point fixation allows for a strong and sound reconstruction of the disorder. The septal flaps are routinely stitched back together with a quilting stitch of 4-0 plain gut suture to avoid hematoma, preclude the need for packing, and further reinforce the stability of the septum.

In cases of alar collapse on inspiration, the cephalic turn-in flap of the LLC or alar batten grafts are useful techniques for reconstruction.[10,25,26] Each of these techniques is aimed at increasing the strength of the LLCs so that they may resist collapse on forced nasal inspiration. The cephalic turn-in flap is especially useful in cases when cephalic trim is necessary to narrow the tip aesthetically and when other graft materials like septal cartilage are in short supply.[25,26]

For turn-in flaps, the cephalic border of the LLC that is planned for excision is scored rather than removed (Video 2). Scoring allows one to fold the cartilage under the remaining LLC, thereby strengthening and straightening the LLC. The turn-in flap is fixed with sutures that are long-lasting or permanent. Mucosa must be underlined partially off the undersurface of the cephalic part of the LLC to allow the cartilage to turn in. Also, a small notch of about 1 mm^2 should be excised at the medial aspect of the turn-in flap to allow easier movement and prevent tip distortion (**Fig. 14**A–F).

Alar batten grafts can be placed intranasally through a small marginal incision and laid over the LLC, while extending to the pyriform aperture.[10] Through an external

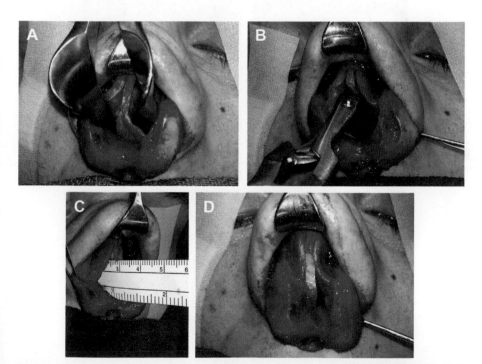

Fig. 13. (*A*) Caudal septal deformity causing static nasal valve obstruction viewed after ULCs have been separated to improve access. (*B*) The caudal end has been resected above the nasal valve angle. (*C*) Measuring the depth of the caudal end for the replacement graft. (*D*) The caudal end has been replaced and is partially fixated to the ULCs and the dorsal septal remnant with 5-0 PDS suture in a figure-of-eight and to the nasal spine with a 3-0 monocryl Wright suture.

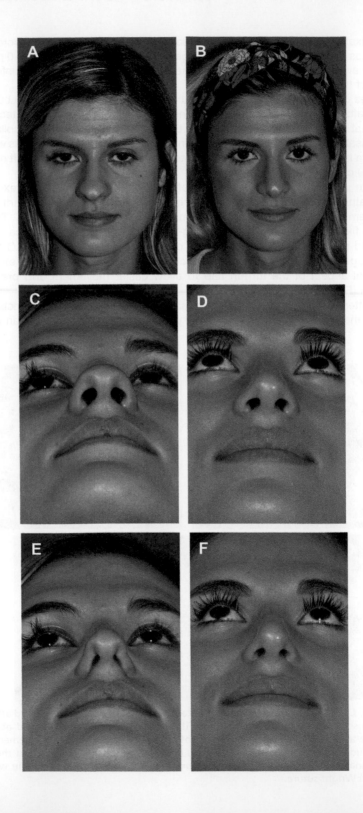

approach, they can be placed either above or below the layer of the LLCs or extend out to the pyriform aperture. In either case, the marginal incision should taper inferiorly to the LLC from halfway down the LLC to the pyriform aperture to allow easier graft placement and fixation.

The underlay technique is especially useful in very bulbous tips when freeing the LLCs to the dome allows the surgeon to optimally reshape the cartilage into a more aesthetically pleasing manner. Permanent or long-lasting sutures are essential in fixating grafts placed through the external approach. Otherwise, the contractile forces of the healing skin and soft tissue envelope will inevitably shift the graft.

The surgeon can mark the point of maximal collapse with the patient awake. A suction test can be applied intraoperatively before starting surgery.[27] The suction tip is applied to 1 nostril while the other nostril is obstructed with the thumb. The point of maximal collapse will be apparent and can be marked. After closure of the nose, the collapse can be reassessed for evaluating the security and success of the surgeon's grafting techniques.

THE CROOKED NOSE

The crooked nose is more common in European and Caucasian noses than in other ethnic groups because of the higher dorsum usually present in this group. The crooked nose can result from a bony, a cartilaginous, or a combination deformity.[14] Many times the crooked nose is a result of nasal trauma.[14,18] However, many patients have a crooked nose congenitally. The nose must be carefully assessed preoperatively to determine whether the issue is mainly bony, mainly cartilaginous, or a combination of both.

Bony deformities are typically addressed with osteotomies to correct the distorted bony pyramid.[15] Many times a combination of osteotomies is necessary. The most common combination used in this author's practice to correct the bony dorsum is complete bilateral lateral osteotomies and an intermediate osteotomy on the longer, flatter side of the nasal bone. These osteotomies may be combined with an outfracturing medial osteotomy on the longer, flatter side of the bone. Typically, osteotomies are started medially and progress laterally to maintain stability of the nose during the procedure (**Fig. 15**A-F).

Cartilaginous asymmetry may be partially or completely corrected with the osteotomies alone. However, in many cases, some level of cartilaginous manipulation is necessary to correct abnormalities of the cartilaginous nose. Septoplasty, caudal end transplant, dome divisions, tip grafts, spreader grafts, batten grafts, alar struts, and sidewall onlays are all common techniques to correct the deviated cartilaginous nose (**Fig. 15**). Because these techniques are vast, the reader is referred to general rhinoplasty textbooks and the references cited in this article for a more in-depth presentation of the techniques.

Fig. 14. (*A*) A patient with a dorsal bump, bulbous nasal tip, dynamic nasal valve collapse, and a straight septum. (*B*) The same patient 1 year after cephalic turn in flaps, dorsal bump resection, lateral osteotomies, tip placation, and stabilization sutures. (*C*) Base view at rest before surgery. (*D*) Base view at rest after surgery. (*E*) Base view with forced nasal inspiration demonstrates severe dynamic nasal valve collapse. (*F*) Base view after surgery on forced nasal inspiration shows resolution of dynamic nasal valve collapse.

252

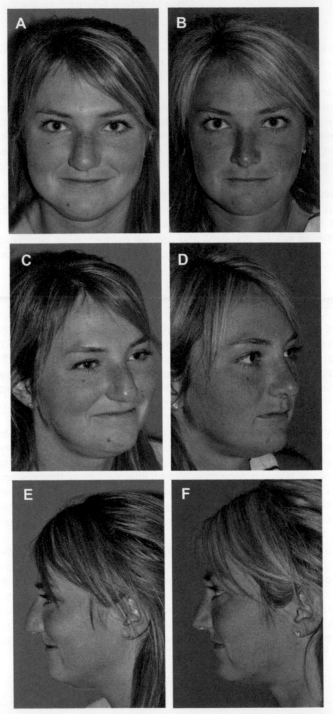

Fig. 15. (*A*) A patient with a wide, ill-defined nasal tip, crooked nose, and dorsal bump. (*B*) Five months after septorhinoplasty, with bump excision, left intermediate osteotomy, bilateral complete lateral osteotomies, cephalic turn in flaps, dome plication sutures, crushed cartilage radix graft, columellar strut, fat removal between the medial crural feet, and a morselized shield tip graft. (*C*) Three-quarter view before. (*D*) Three-quarter view after. (*E*) Lateral view before. (*F*) Lateral view after.

SUMMARY

The European or Caucasian nose presents multiple unique challenges for the rhinoplasty surgeon. Many of these problems and options for repair are presented in this article. Certainly a multitude of other techniques are available beyond those presented. Rhinoplasty is an exciting surgery, and the surgeon learns through his or her lifetime of experience and exposure to new techniques.

DISCLOSURES

None.

SUPPLEMENTARY DATA

Supplementary data related to this article can be found online at https://doi.org/10.1016/j.otc.2019.12.003.

REFERENCES

1. Bhopal R, Donaldson L. White, European, Western, Caucasian or what? Inappropriate labeling in research on race, ethnicity, and health. Am J Public Health 1998;88(9):1303–7.
2. Johnson CM Jr, Toriumi DM. Open structure rhinoplasty. Philadelphia: W B Saunders Co; 1990.
3. Whitaker EG, Johnson CM Jr. The evolution of open structure rhinoplasty. Arch Facial Plast Surg 2003;5(4):291–300.
4. Anderson JR. A reasoned approach to nasal base surgery. Arch Otolaryngol 1984;110(6):349–58.
5. Janeke JB, Wright WK. Studies in the support of the nasal tip. Arch Otolaryngol 1971;93(5):458–64.
6. Gassner HG, Remington WJ, Sherris DA. Quantitative studies of nasal tip support and the effect of reconstructive rhinoplasty. Arch Facial Plast Surg 2001;(3):178–84.
7. Westreich RW, Lawson W. The tripod theory of nasal tip support revisited: the cantilevered spring model. Arch Facial Plast Surg 2008;10(3):170–9.
8. Khurana D, Sherris DA. Grafting materials for augmentation septorhinoplasty. Facial Plast Surg 1999;7(4):210–6.
9. Kridel RWH, Scott BA, Foda HMT. The tongue-and-groove technique in septorhinoplasty. A ten-year experience. Arch Facial Plast Surg 1999;1(4):246–56.
10. Toriumi DM, Josen J, Weinberger N, et al. Use of alar batten grafts for correction of nasal valve collapse. Operative Tech Otolaryngol Head Neck Surg 1995;6(4):311–9.
11. Sherris DA, Oriel DS. Acellular human dermal matrix in rhinoplasty. Aesthet Surg J 2011;31(7):95S–100S.
12. Johnson CM Jr, Godin MS. The tension nose: open structure rhinoplasty approach. Plast Reconstr Surg 1995;95(1):43–51.
13. Wurm J, Kovacebic M. A new classification of spreader flap technique. Facial Plast Surg 2013;29:506–14.
14. Kienstra MA, Gassner HG, Sherris DA, et al. A grading system for nasal dorsal deformities. Arch Facial Plast Surg 2003;5:138–43.
15. Kienstra MA, Sherris DA, Kern EB. Osteotomy in pyramid modification in the Joseph and Cottle rhinoplasty. Facial Plast Surg Clin North Am 1999;7(3):279–94.

16. Gassner HZ, Friedman O, Sherris DA, et al. An alternative method of middle valve reconstruction. Arch Facial Plast Surg 2006;8(6):432–5.
17. Saban Y, Daniel RK, Polselli R, et al. Dorsal preservation: the push-down technique reassessed. Aesthet Surg J 2008;38(2):117–31.
18. Wei JR, Remington WJ, Sherris DA. Evaluation of patients with nasal obstruction. Facial Plast Surg 1999;(7):263–78.
19. Kern EB. Surgical approaches to abnormalities of the nasal valve. Rhinology 1978;16:165–89.
20. Goode RL. Surgery of the incompetent nasal valve. Laryngoscope 1985;(95):546–55.
21. Sherris DA. Caudal and dorsal septal reconstruction: an algorithm for graft choices. Am J Rhinol 1997;11:457–66.
22. Sherris DA, Kern EB. Versatile autogenous rib graft in septorhinoplasty. Am J Rhinol 1998;12(3):221–7.
23. Sherris DA. The versatile autogenous costal cartilage graft in septorhinoplasty–commentary. Arch Facial Plast Surg 2002;4(2):177–9.
24. Williams CT, Sherris DA. Caudal septal reconstruction for severe deviation: a modification to respect the valve area. Am Otolaryng Rhino 2016;3(4):1097.
25. Tellioglu AP, Cimen K. Turn-in folding of the cephalic portion of the lateral crus to support the alar rim in rhinoplasty. Aesthetic Plast Surg 2007;31(3):306–10.
26. Murakami CS, Barrera JE, Most FP. Preserving structural integrity of the alar cartilage in aesthetic rhinoplasty with a turn-In Flap. Arch Facial Plast Surg 2009;11(2):126–8.
27. Zoumalan RA, Larrabee WF Jr, Murakami CS. Intraoperative functional evaluation of the nasal valve in rhinoplasty. Arch Facial Plast Surg 2012;14(1):34–8.

Use of Nasal Implants and Dorsal Modification When Treating the East Asian Nose

Hyung Gyun Na, MD[a], Yong Ju Jang, MD, PhD[b],*

KEYWORDS

- Asian rhinoplasty • Dorsal augmentation • Alloplastic material • Autologous material

KEY POINTS

- The goal of rhinoplasty in most East Asians is the augmentation of the nasal dorsum and tip.
- In Asian rhinoplasty, alloplastic material, such as silicone and Gore-Tex, are widely used implants in patients who desire to have a high dorsum and well-projected tip.
- In the case of minimal correction and augmentation, injection of filler can be a useful option.
- Autologous materials, like septal cartilage, conchal cartilage, costal cartilage, and dermo-fat, have benefits, such as lower risk of infection and better long-term functional outcomes.
- These materials may hold distinct disadvantages over others when one considers tissue availability, donor site morbidity, and additional operative time.

ANATOMIC CHARACTERISTICS AND PREFERRED SHAPE OF THE EAST ASIAN NOSE

Dorsal augmentation is the most essential component of rhinoplasty for East Asians. It is crucial not only in simple cosmetic rhinoplasty but also in all other types for aesthetic perfection. Correct augmentation is determined by the height and shape of the nasal dorsum observed from the side and front, and the harmonious alignment with the nasal tip. Compared with Caucasian nose shapes, the East Asian noses tend to have a broad and flat nasal dorsum with an underprojected tip.

The ideal ratio of the Caucasian nose, on average, is 2:1:1:0.75 for length, projection, height, and radix, respectively.[1] A study of young Korean individuals reported those measurements to be different; they have a nasal length-to-tip projection to

[a] Department of Otorhinolaryngology–Head and Neck Surgery, University of Yeungnam Cllege of Medicine, 170, Hyeonchung-ro, Nam-gu, Daegu, Korea; [b] Department of Otolaryngology, Asan Medical Center, University of Ulsan College of Medicine, 86 Asanbyeongwon-gil, Songpa-gu, Seoul 05505, South Korea
* Corresponding author.
E-mail address: jangyj@amc.seoul.kr

Otolaryngol Clin N Am 53 (2020) 255–266
https://doi.org/10.1016/j.otc.2019.12.004
0030-6665/20/© 2019 Elsevier Inc. All rights reserved.
oto.theclinics.com

dorsal height-to-radix height ratio of 2:0.97:0.61:0.28.[2] These data indicate that East Asians have lower dorsal and radix heights.

Regarding the shape of the nasal dorsum, 67.2% of Asians preferred the straight type; 29.7% preferred the middle concave type, and the remaining preferred the mildly convex type. Particularly, men preferred the straight type for the dorsal line, and women preferred the mild concave type.[3] Dorsal lines in women, as seen from the side, may preferably be placed a little lower than the line connecting the nasofrontal angle and tip, in a slightly concave shape. In male patients, to avoid a feminine appearance, the dorsal line should be placed on or slightly above the nasofrontal angle-tip line. In female East Asian patients, the nasion or nasal starting point should be placed at a level between the midpupillary and double eyelid lines, considering the patient's preferred nose shape. In male patients, it may be preferable to place the nasion slightly higher.

Considering the shape of the tip, a double break consisting of both the supratip and the infratip breaks is considered ideal in Caucasians; however, the thicker skin of East Asians make it exceedingly difficult to obtain the double break. Specifically, to produce a good tip definition from the low and round lower lateral cartilage (LLC), it is necessary to ensure that the LLC has anterocaudal projections. In addition, cephalic malposition was seen as the cause for the formation of the bulbous tip in Westerners, but according to the authors' study, cephalic malposition was not as definitely evident in East Asians with a bulbous tip. In fact, because of a thicker skin, and smaller and weaker LLC causing the formation of a sufficient tip projection to be difficult, East Asians tend to have underprojected tips.[4]

SILICONE

Patients who pursue dorsal augmentation generally desire excellent results with prompt recovery without significant morbidity. In that regard, a silicone implant is the ideal choice for many surgeons because it has a smooth surface, no dorsal irregularity, and no volume changes over time, is easy to design, and brings excellent aesthetic results. Thus, it is the most commonly used implant material in Asia. One of the reasons for favorable outcomes using silicone implants is that Asians have thicker skin tissue than Caucasians; thus, they have lower risks of complications, such as implant extrusion.[5] There are many additional advantages of silicone that made this material the most popular implant: excellent biocompatibility, availability in various levels of hardness, low cost, and ease of removal when problems occur. In order for it to be used as a dorsal implant, a canoe-shaped silicone implant is designed, and the caudal end of the implant is carved in a sharp, angulated shape to fit the cephalic divergence of the alar cartilages and is fixed to the surrounding cartilage tissue using sutures. The commonly selected implants are those with 2 to 5 mm thickness. Although many different forms of prefabricated silicone implants are available, they will not correspond to every different style of individual noses, necessitating personalized carving in each patient before and during operation.[6] An L-shaped silicone is used to raise both the nasal tip and the dorsum using silicone. When using the L-shaped implant, if the surgeon applies greater tension on the tip to achieve a tent-pole effect, the skin of the nasal tip could become too thin in the long term.

There are problems related to the use of silicone in dorsal augmentation, despite its ease in creating a smooth dorsal contour. Extrusion (2%–4%), infection (4%), and displacement (3%) have been reported as possible complications, but the results have varied depending on the skills and expertise of the surgeon.[7] Infection is one of the most serious complications; erythema, swelling, and purulent discharge are typical signs. Delayed infection can also be a problem that often presents as recurrent swelling and mild erythema, where the formation of a bacterial biofilm on the implant surface may be related.[8] Aesthetically improper implant design is also a common complication. Capsule formation, skin contraction, telangiectasia, and chronic recurrent inflammation are other frequent complications. Silicone can cause dorsal irregularity through calcification of the silicone, which becomes much more extensive in the long term, within the nasal dorsum.[9]

One of the most common unpredictable and severe complications that may arise from silicone implantation is short nose deformity.[10] After insertion of silicone, resorption of the nasal cartilage framework that develops over time and contracture of the capsule surrounding the implant can lead to a short nose. As a result of the loss of elasticity and severe fibrosis of the skin soft tissue envelope, corrective surgery for short nose is one of the most difficult reconstructive challenges. To prevent complications, thorough sterilization of the surgical field is necessary for reducing infection, especially in the nasal vestibule and the nasal cavity. During surgery, it is important to prevent breakage of the natural barrier, such as a mucous membrane injury. In cases that involve a significant modification of the normal anatomic structure like osteotomies, infection is a chief concern.

Efforts are being made to reduce complications of silicone rhinoplasty, mostly the combined use of biologic tissue and silicone. Suh and colleagues[11] reported that the concomitant use of acellular dermal matrix and silicone has the potential to correct visibility of silicone implants and significantly decrease capsule thickness and myofibroblast activity. Agrawal and colleagues[12] also reported that the ride-on technique, where the autologous materials such as cartilage or perichondrium is sutured onto the surface of silicone, maintains natural mobility of the tip and reduces implant extrusion rates.

Dorsal augmentation using silicone is an essential component of Asian rhinoplasty and can bring about excellent aesthetic outcomes with relative ease. To obtain the best results using silicone implants, meticulous surgical planning and aesthetically appropriate implant design are crucial, along with mastery of the various tip surgery techniques.

GORE-TEX

Gore-Tex (expanded polytetrafluoroethylene [ePTFE]; W.L. Gore and Associates, Flagstaff, AZ, USA) is a porous material; the holes of the ePTFE are filled with various types of cells, such as those in connective tissues, fibrous tissue, collagen, and capillary vessels, causing the material to be firmly fixed to the surrounding tissues. The advantage of using ePTFE is that the material is not as rigid as silicone, has a softer texture that decreases the patient's discomfort after insertion into the nasal dorsum, and allows the nose to look more natural. From the surgeon's perspective, the major disadvantage associated with using Gore-Tex is that it is more difficult to carve than silicone because of its softer physical property, and it shows a possibility of decreasing volume in human tissue over time.[13] Furthermore, in procedures whereby a greater amount of dorsal augmentation is necessary, the need to overlay several layers of the material increases the complexity of shaping the implant.

The Surgiform (Surgiform, Columbia, SC, USA) implant, made up of reinforced ePTFE, is available in various prefabricated shapes that meet the needs of the surgeon, much like silicone implants (**Fig. 1**).[14]

In the senior author's previous study, when aesthetic outcomes and complications of using ePTFE and autologous cartilage were compared, dorsal augmentation using ePTFE represented similar aesthetic outcomes and lower complication rates.[15]

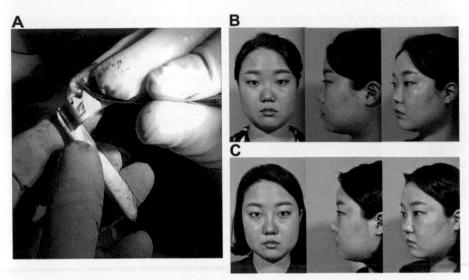

Fig. 1. Patient with an improved dorsal aesthetic line and augmented nasal dorsum by using a prefabricated ePTFE implant. (*A*) Intraoperative modification of the undersurface of the implant with a razor blade. (*B*) Preoperative photograph. (*C*) Postoperative photograph.

A different form of Gore-Tex implant, Sili-Tex (Wish, Taipei, Taiwan), is made of an inner silicone core with the outer surface wrapped with ePTFE. The inner silicone core helps to maintain a constant height, and the outer ePTFE reduces implant mobility by ingrowth of the neighboring tissue.[16] This silicone-polytetrafluoroethylene composite implant has biocompatibility and minimal foreign body reaction.[17]

With the increasing use of Gore-Tex, complications, such as extrusion, uneven surface, infection, recurrent swelling, and seroma, have also been increasingly reported.[18,19] Bai and colleagues[20] suggest that the double "V" carving technique may be applied to enhance nasal dynamic mobility. In their technique, a bilateral wedge incision is made at the junction of the mobile and fixed parts of the nasal dorsum. The angle of incision is 25° to 45°, and the width is one-third of the prosthesis' width.

INJECTABLE FILLER

When compared with standard rhinoplasty using allograft and autologous grafts, injectable filler is less invasive, simple, effective, and cost-effective. It is the second most commonly performed cosmetic procedure globally and mainly performed for augmentation of the nasal dorsum and radix in the Asian nose. The selection of patients is important for successful postoperative results. Good candidates of filler injection in the Asian nose are patients who have a minor hump, minor deviations, a high nasal tip and low nasal dorsum, or a slight irregularity.

The ingredients of fillers widely vary from autologous fat, collagen, hyaluronic acid, calcium hydroxylapatite, paraffin, and liquid silicone. To minimize dorsal distortion or deviation after injection, multiple site injections rather than a single-point injection should be performed to fill the whole length of the nasal dorsum along the straight dorsal line.[21] The ideal and safe location of injection in nasal dorsum is in the avascular plane. Most literature suggests the layer of filler injection area lies between the superficial musculoaponeurotic system and perichondrium or periosteum.[22]

Although injection rhinoplasty is relatively safe and less traumatic, typical postoperative complications, including swelling, erythema, bruising, and asymmetry, may develop. Furthermore, the probability of rather drastic vascular complications, like skin necrosis, blindness, and cerebral infarction, should be taken into account seriously.[23,24] These vascular complications can be a consequence of either intravascular injection or the compressive effect of the filler on peripheral vessels.[25] Although there are no definitive preventive measures for vascular compromise by filler injections, the following are the instructions to help the surgeon minimize complications[21,22,26]:

1. One should be familiar with the vascular anatomy of the nose.
2. Aspiration should be performed before filler injection.
3. Small and blunt needles or cannulas should be used.
4. The smallest volume should be injected at a low pressure.
5. One has to be vigilant on the development of several typical symptoms, such as initial toothache and headache, which indicate that the filler has been injected into an artery.
6. The surgeon should be prepared for severe complications by having on hand nitroglycerin paste, hyaluronidase, and systemic or topical steroids, to be used immediately when there is concern for the development of various complications, such as nodules, erythema, skin necrosis, and visual impairment.

AUTOLOGOUS IMPLANTS

The most commonly used autologous materials for dorsal augmentation are septal cartilage, conchal cartilage, costal cartilage, dermofat, and fascia.

SEPTAL CARTILAGE

East Asian noses have not only less septal cartilage but also weak septal framework. According to the senior author's study, the average septal cartilage harvested during external rhinoplasty, leaving an L-strut of 1 cm, has a caudal length, dorsal length, and area of 15.1 mm, 18.2 mm, and 520.9 mm^2, respectively.[27]

The septal cartilage in the Asian nose is commonly used for structural modification, including a columellar strut, spreader graft, septal extension graft, and tip grafts, such as an onlay graft, shield graft, and multilayer tip graft. After using septal cartilage in the aforementioned procedures, in most cases, only a small amount of septal cartilage remains. The authors believe that the use of septal cartilage for dorsal augmentation is not an ideal surgical option. First, it is difficult to obtain a sufficiently long piece of septal cartilage (3–4 cm) for dorsal augmentation. Second, using a septal cartilage with an angled margin for dorsal augmentation is less aesthetically suitable compared with using alloplastic implants. Thus, it is uncommon to use septal cartilage as a 1-piece dorsal augmentation material. Usually, the piece of cartilage that remains after structural grafting or tip grafting is crushed using a cartilage crusher and used as a volume filler to correct focal depressions or uneven areas in the nasal dorsum or tip (Fig. 2).

To overcome the insufficient amount of septal cartilage for dorsal augmentation, Harel and Margulis[28] reported the effectiveness of diced septal cartilage enclosed with temporalis fascia for dorsal augmentation in the Asian nose.

CONCHAL CARTILAGE

Conchal cartilage possesses similar characteristics to that of the LLC, making it suitable for nasal tip augmentation. However, because of its intrinsic curvature and

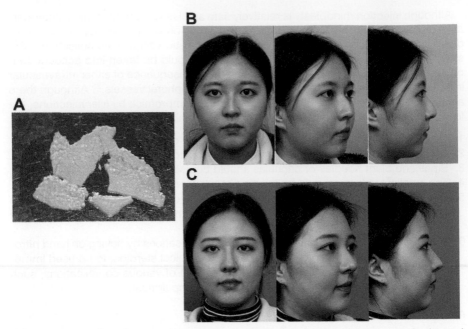

Fig. 2. Patient with an improved tip shape as a result of tip grafting by using crushed septal cartilage. (*A*) Intraoperative photograph of a prepared crushed septal cartilage for dorsal augmentation. (*B*) Preoperative photograph, and (*C*) postoperative photograph.

limitations in length, conchal cartilage has clear limitations as dorsal augmentation material. For full-length nasal augmentation using conchal cartilage alone, from the radix to the tip, one must harvest a large piece of cartilage. In such cases, its natural curvature can be eliminated by cutting it in a convex shape and stacking it into multiple layers.[29] However, dorsal augmentation using such methods increases the possibility of contour visibility of the graft through the skin over time. Therefore, the use of a diced conchal cartilage wrapped with various materials is a popular way of using ear cartilage for dorsal augmentation. Erol[30] reported that diced conchal cartilage graft wrapped in Surgicel (Johnson & Johnson, New Brunswick, NJ, USA) is suitable for dorsal augmentation. Daniel[31] modified its application by use of diced cartilage graft wrapped in temporalis fascia. This method has been a widely accepted procedure in the past decade because of an ease of preparation and decreased resorption rate. Varedi and Bohluli[32] introduced a composite graft consisting of conchal cartilage and retroauricular fascia. The senior author of this article reported the usefulness of diced conchal cartilage with that of an intact perichondrium for dorsal augmentation, especially for segmental augmentation (**Fig. 3**).[33]

In addition, there are some studies on the utility of autologous tissue glue, such as fibrin glue and whole blood. Tasman[34] emphasized the usefulness of diced cartilage in fibrin glue graft, which had lower resorption rate and provided favorable aesthetic outcomes. Codazzi and colleagues[35] reported that the mixture of diced cartilage and warm blood is also an extremely convenient and easy technique for dorsal augmentation. The disadvantages of using conchal cartilage are insufficient amount for substantial augmentation and likelihood of donor site morbidity, such as hematoma and keloid formation. Recipient site complications, such as graft resorption, infection, and dorsal irregularity, may also develop.[36]

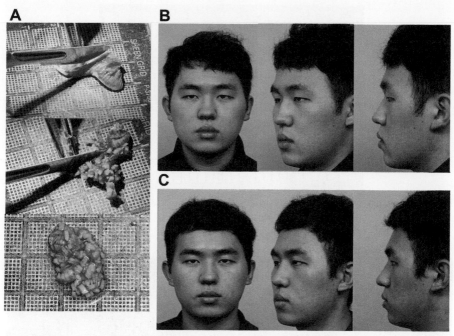

Fig. 3. Patient with a saddle nose deformity was treated with a diced conchal cartilage with intact perichondrium for dorsal augmentation. (*A*) Intraoperative photograph of a prepared diced conchal cartilage for dorsal augmentation. (*B*) Preoperative photograph, and (*C*) postoperative photograph.

COSTAL CARTILAGE

The use of costal cartilage is becoming increasingly popular in Asian rhinoplasty in recent years. Costal cartilage is a versatile material that can be used for dorsal augmentation as well as modification of the nasal tip and septal reconstruction. Costal cartilage is inarguably the best material when the surgeon needs ample graft material in nasal reconstruction. The authors use costal cartilage for the following conditions: reconstructive rhinoplasty that requires large amounts of sturdy cartilage for nasal septal reconstruction and grafting owing to severe deformation; saddle nose; short nose; the patient who has a small nose and wants major changes; and when the patient with very thick skin wants well-defined and projected nasal tips with distinct contour.

The most frequently recommended method of using rib cartilage for dorsal augmentation is to shape a 3- to 4-cm monoblock implant, especially when a substantial augmentation of greater than 5 mm is required (**Fig. 4**). Carving of the costal cartilage block well is important, but extremely difficult and tedious. An implant must be meticulously carved to well fit the underlying nasal skeleton. To prevent an unexpected deviation of the costal cartilage implant, the skin pocket should tightly fit the size of the graft. Moreover, it is better to suture-fixate the graft to the upper lateral cartilages and cephalic end of the lateral crus. K-wire fixation through the skin, graft, and underlying nasal bone is a different way of graft stabilization.[31] However, in creating a natural-looking and smooth dorsum, successful 1-piece dorsal augmentation using rib cartilage for the entire dorsum is extremely difficult and requires considerable experience (**Fig. 5**). Aesthetic complications, such as warping, implant visibility, contour

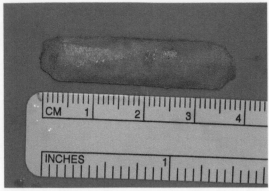

Fig. 4. Monoblock costal cartilage approximately 3.5 cm in size for dorsal augmentation.

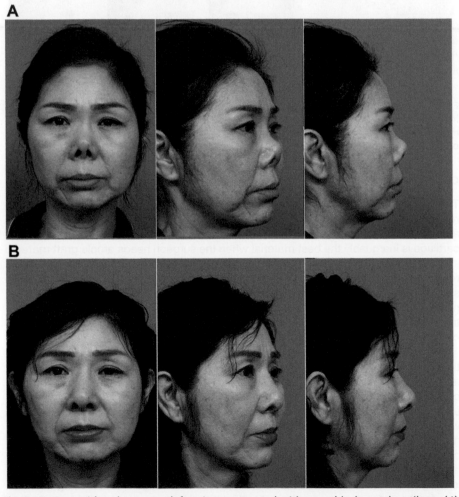

Fig. 5. Patient with a short nose deformity was treated with monoblock costal cartilage. (*A*) Preoperative photograph, and (*B*) postoperative photograph.

irregularity, graft mobility, and resorption of the dorsal implant, commonly occur.[37] Because of the shrink-wrap phenomenon, in the long-term follow-up of the patient, especially in the thin-skinned individual, there is high risk of developing prominent contour of the cartilage graft. The authors, therefore, do not recommend using costal cartilage as a nasal dorsal implant unless there are no other choices.

In order to overcome the drawbacks of dorsal augmentation using solid block costal cartilage, different ways of using the costal cartilage for nasal dorsum have been introduced. Diced cartilage wrapped with temporalis fascia grafts has been widely accepted in the past decade because of the ease of preparation, and several other advantages, such as no risk of warping, good survival rate of graft, and maximizing the usage of harvested cartilage.[31] Cerkes and Basaran[38] showed that the rectus abdominis fascia can be used to eliminate additional donor site through the same incision during costal cartilage harvest. Instead of using temporalis fascia, which induces harvesting morbidity, the use of alternative wrapping materials, such as Tutoplast (RTI Surgical, Marquette, MI, USA) -processed fascia lata and Alloderm (Biohorizons, Birmingham, AL, USA), has also been suggested.[39,40] Although the diced cartilage wrapped with fascia or other materials is easier to shape into a natural-looking nasal dorsum compared with the use of solid block (**Fig. 6**), this method is not free from complications, such as graft deviation, dorsal irregularity or focal depression, resorption, and visibility of diced cartilage particle through the skin. To prevent inherent problems with wrapping material, Bullocks and colleagues[41] reported that the use of autologous tissue glue to stabilize diced costal cartilage is an acceptable technique for dorsal augmentation. However, this technique has a potential risk of manifesting dorsal irregularity, and it is difficult to deliver the glued diced cartilage to the nasal dorsum. Free diced costal cartilage without wrapping material also can be used as a camouflage graft and requires minor augmentation, improving dorsal irregularities in the Asian nose.[42] Tan and colleagues[43–46] introduced the usefulness of a

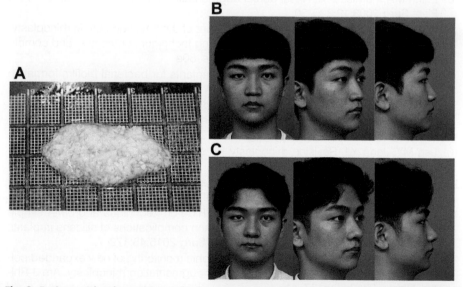

Fig. 6. Patient with a favorable aesthetic dorsal augmentation after the graft of using diced costal cartilage. (*A*) Intraoperative photograph of a prepared diced costal cartilage for dorsal augmentation. (*B*) Preoperative photograph, and (*C*) postoperative photograph.

"sandwich" graft for saddle nose correction, which is placing the costal cartilage block beneath a dermal fat graft.

SUMMARY

The choice of dorsal implant material is influenced by the needs and conditions of the patients, the material preference skills, and the experience of the surgeon. All materials have pros and cons, so there is no single ideal implant or graft for dorsal augmentation. For successful results, a thorough understanding of the shape of an aesthetically perfect nose, proper surgical technique, and technical management methods for complications are needed.

DISCLOSURE

The authors have nothing to disclose.

REFERENCES

1. Mowlavi A, Wilhelmi BJ. A clinical definition of an ideal nasal radix. Plast Reconstr Surg 2003;111:943–4.
2. Wang JH, Jang YJ, Park SK, et al. Measurement of aesthetic proportions in the profile view of Koreans. Ann Plast Surg 2009;62:109–13.
3. Yu MS, Jang YJ. Preoperative computer simulation for Asian rhinoplasty patients: analysis of accuracy and patient preference. Aesthet Surg J 2014;34:1162–71.
4. Na HG, Jang YJ. Intraoperative measurement of the anatomic features of the lower lateral cartilage and nasal tip shape of the Asian nose. JAMA Facial Plast Surg 2018;20:518–9.
5. Jang YJ, Yu MS. Rhinoplasty for the Asian nose. Facial Plast Surg 2010;26: 93–101.
6. Erlich MA, Parhiscar A. Nasal dorsal augmentation with silicone implants. Facial Plast Surg 2003;19:325–30.
7. Lee MR, Unger JG, Rohrich RJ. Management of the nasal dorsum in rhinoplasty: a systematic review of the literature regarding technique, outcomes, and complications. Plast Reconstr Surg 2011;128:538e–50e.
8. Walker TJ, Toriumi DM. Analysis of facial implants for bacterial biofilm formation using scanning electron microscopy. JAMA Facial Plast Surg 2016;18:299–304.
9. Jung DH, Kim BR, Choi JY, et al. Gross and pathologic analysis of long-term silicone implants inserted into the human body for augmentation rhinoplasty: 221 revision cases. Plast Reconstr Surg 2007;120:1997–2003.
10. Lan MY, Jang YJ. Revision rhinoplasty for short noses in the Asian population. JAMA Facial Plast Surg 2015;17:325–32.
11. Suh MK, Lee KH, Harijan A, et al. Augmentation rhinoplasty with silicone implant covered with acellular dermal matrix. J Craniofac Surg 2017;28:445–8.
12. Agrawal KS, Bachhav MV, Naik CS, et al. "Ride-on" technique and other simple and logical solutions to counter most common complications of silicone implants in augmentation rhinoplasty. Indian J Plast Surg 2015;48:172–7.
13. Jung YG, Kim KH, Dhong HJ. Ultrasonographic monitoring of new expanded polytetrafluoroethylene implant thickness after augmentation rhinoplasty. Am J Rhinol Allergy 2012;26:e137–41.
14. Lee SJ, Rho BI, Nam SM, et al. Changes in implant thickness after rhinoplasty using surgiform. Arch Aesthetic Plast Surg 2018;24:1–5.

15. Joo YH, Jang YJ. Comparison of the surgical outcomes of dorsal augmentation using expanded polytetrafluoroethylene or autologous costal cartilage. JAMA Facial Plast Surg 2016;18:327–32.
16. Nguyen AH, Bartlett EL, Kania K, et al. Simple implant augmentation rhinoplasty. Semin Plast Surg 2015;29:247–54.
17. Zelken JA, Hong JP, Chang CS, et al. Silicone-polytetrafluoroethylene composite implants for Asian rhinoplasty. Ann Plast Surg 2017;78:131–7.
18. Ham J, Miller PJ. Expanded polytetrafluoroethylene implants in rhinoplasty: literature review, operative techniques, and outcome. Facial Plast Surg 2003;19:331–9.
19. Yap EC, Abubakar SS, Olveda MB. Expanded polytetrafluoroethylene as dorsal augmentation material in rhinoplasty on Southeast Asian noses: three-year experience. Arch Facial Plast Surg 2011;13:234–8.
20. Bai SS, Li D, Xu L, et al. A novel method to enhance dynamic rhinoplasty outcomes: double "V" carving for alloplastic grafts. Ear Nose Throat J 2019. https://doi.org/10.1177/0145561319840110. 145561319840110.
21. Tansatit T, Moon HJ, Rungsawang C, et al. Safe planes for injection rhinoplasty: a histological analysis of midline longitudinal sections of the Asian nose. Aesthetic Plast Surg 2016;40:236–44.
22. Moon HJ. Injection rhinoplasty using filler. Facial Plast Surg Clin North Am 2018;26:323–30.
23. Kim EG, Eom TK, Kang SJ. Severe visual loss and cerebral infarction after injection of hyaluronic acid gel. J Craniofac Surg 2014;25:684–6.
24. Cohen E, Yatziv Y, Leibovitch I, et al. A case report of ophthalmic artery emboli secondary to calcium hydroxylapatite filler injection for nose augmentation–long-term outcome. BMC Ophthalmol 2016;16:98.
25. Chen QQ, Liu Y, Fan DL. Serious vascular complications after nonsurgical rhinoplasty: a case report. Plast Reconstr Surg Glob Open 2016;4:e683.
26. Bertossi D, Giampaoli G, Verner I, et al. Complications and management after a nonsurgical rhinoplasty: a literature review. Dermatol Ther 2019;32:e12978.
27. Kim JS, Khan NA, Song HM, et al. Intraoperative measurements of harvestable septal cartilage in rhinoplasty. Ann Plast Surg 2010;65:519–23.
28. Harel M, Margulis A. Dorsal augmentation with diced cartilage enclosed with temporal fascia in secondary endonasal rhinoplasty. Aesthet Surg J 2013;33:809–16.
29. Hagerty RC, Mittelstaedt S, Vu LP, et al. Countercurve placement of conchal cartilage grafts used for correction of nasal tip deformities. Ann Plast Surg 2007;59:566–8.
30. Erol OO. The Turkish delight: a pliable graft for rhinoplasty. Plast Reconstr Surg 2000;105:2229–41.
31. Daniel RK. Diced cartilage grafts in rhinoplasty surgery: current techniques and applications. Plast Reconstr Surg 2008;122:1883–91.
32. Varedi P, Bohluli B. Dorsal nasal augmentation: is the composite graft consisting of conchal cartilage and retroauricular fascia an effective option? J Oral Maxillofac Surg 2015;73:1842.e1-13.
33. Kim JH, Jang YJ. Use of diced conchal cartilage with perichondrial attachment in rhinoplasty. Plast Reconstr Surg 2015;135:1545–53.
34. Tasman AJ, Suarez GA. The diced cartilage glue graft for radix augmentation in rhinoplasty. JAMA Facial Plast Surg 2015;17:303–4.
35. Codazzi D, Ortelli L, Robotti E. Diced cartilage combined with warm blood glue for nasal dorsum enhancement. Aesthetic Plast Surg 2014;38:822–3.

36. Lan MY, Park JP, Jang YJ. Donor site morbidities resulting from conchal cartilage harvesting in rhinoplasty. J Laryngol Otol 2017;131:529–33.
37. Moon BJ, Lee HJ, Jang YJ. Outcomes following rhinoplasty using autologous costal cartilage. Arch Facial Plast Surg 2012;14:175–80.
38. Cerkes N, Basaran K. Diced cartilage grafts wrapped in rectus abdominis fascia for nasal dorsum augmentation. Plast Reconstr Surg 2016;137:43–51.
39. Jang YJ, Song HM, Yoon YJ, et al. Combined use of crushed cartilage and processed fascia lata for dorsal augmentation in rhinoplasty for Asians. Laryngoscope 2009;119:1088–92.
40. Gordon CR, Alghoul M, Goldberg JS, et al. Diced cartilage grafts wrapped in alloderm for dorsal nasal augmentation. J Craniofac Surg 2011;22:1196–9.
41. Bullocks JM, Echo A, Guerra G, et al. A novel autologous scaffold for diced-cartilage grafts in dorsal augmentation rhinoplasty. Aesthetic Plast Surg 2011;35:569–79.
42. Yoo SH, Jang YJ. Rib cartilage in Asian rhinoplasty: new trends. Curr Opin Otolaryngol Head Neck Surg 2019;27:261–6.
43. Tan O, Algan S, Cinal H, et al. Management of saddle nose deformity using dermal fat and costal cartilage "sandwich" graft: a problem-oriented approach and anthropometric evaluation. J Oral Maxillofac Surg 2016;74:1848.e1–14.
44. Suh MK. Dorsal augmentation using autogenous tissues. Facial Plast Surg Clin North Am 2018;26:295–310.
45. Na DS, Jung SW, Kook KS, et al. Augmentation rhinoplasty with dermofat graft & fat injection. J Korean Soc Plast Reconstr Surg 2011;38:53–62.
46. Kim HK, Rhee SC. Augmentation rhinoplasty using a folded "pure" dermal graft. J Craniofac Surg 2013;24:1758–62.

Management of the Mestizo Nose

Roxana Cobo, MD

KEYWORDS

- Mestizo rhinoplasty • Latino rhinoplasty • Hispanic rhinoplasty
- Thick-skinned rhinoplasty • Ethnic patient • Structural rhinoplasty

KEY POINTS

- Mestizo rhinoplasty patients are mixed-race patients. They are also known as Hispanic or Latino patients.
- Mestizo patients are ethnic patients with mesorrhine nasal characteristics. The underlying osteocartilaginous framework is modest and they frequently have nasal tips with poor projection and rotation.
- A structural rhinoplasty approach is used with mestizo rhinoplasty patients. This means conservative tissue excision, reinforcement of support structures, and structural grafting and suturing techniques.
- In thick-skinned patients, medical and surgical management of the skin–soft tissue envelope is performed to help improve skin texture and skin definition in nasal tip area.

INTRODUCTION

The term "mestizo" means "mixed" in Spanish and it is a term used all over Latin America to describe a person of mixed-race heritage. In Central and South America it means a combination of European and native Indian heritage.[1] The term "mulato" in Spanish is used to describe people with mixed-race ancestry with a white European and black African background. All across Latin America these two terms are used to describe people of mixed-race ancestry. Mestizos are a racial majority in Mexico, Central America, and South America.[2] Mulato's are seen more in areas of the Caribbean and Central and South America where African ancestry is more predominant.

Race and ethnicity are confusing for most people and frequently they are used interchangeably. In general, most dictionaries define ethnicity as part of a person's cultural identity, language, customs, religion, or even nationality. Race is defined by most dictionaries is based on the person's physical characteristics especially skin color. Trying

Department of Otolaryngology, Centro Médico Imbanaco, Carrera 38A #5A-100 Consultorio 222, Cali, Colombia
E-mail address: rcobo@imbanaco.com.co

Otolaryngol Clin N Am 53 (2020) 267–282
https://doi.org/10.1016/j.otc.2019.12.008
0030-6665/20/© 2019 Elsevier Inc. All rights reserved.

oto.theclinics.com

to categorize people into racial or ethnic groups has always had important political and economic implications in all countries around the world.

In medical literature it is frequent to find the terms "Latino," "Hispanic," or "mestizo." The term "Latino" is short for Latinoamericano in Spanish, which means someone coming from any country in Latin America including Brazil. The term "Hispanic" is usually reserved for those people who are coming from Spanish speaking countries of Latin America (this usually excludes Brazil).[3] According to the US Census, Hispanic or Latino refers to a person of Cuban, Mexican, Puerto Rican, South or Central American, or other Spanish culture or origin regardless of race.[4] This concept is a concept of ethnicity and does not take into account race. Hispanics or Latinos today are considered the largest minority group in the United States. In 2004 the term "Latino" was introduced and its use became widespread in 2014. Latino is a gender-neutral neologism, sometimes used instead of Latino or Latina to refer to people of Latin American cultural or racial identity in the United States.

With all this being said, the term "mestizo" is not used in the United States for official purposes and even though most Latin Americans understand and use this term it is not a common term in many other countries. Today mestizos are considered mixed-race people and this term in the medical literature is used interchangeably with Hispanic and Latino. The term "mestizo rhinoplasty" is probably the one that most accurately defines anatomic characteristics in these patients.

MESTIZO NASAL CHARACTERISTICS

It is not uncommon to find articles in the literature trying to classify the mestizo nose into different categories.[5–7] It becomes difficult to classify patients into "types" because mestizo patients are mixed-race patients and therefore innumerable types of noses are seen.

Mestizo characteristics vary from region to region and the changes depend on where the patient is coming from and what predominant race he or she has (white, black, Indian). In general terms, mestizo noses are classified as mesorrhine noses (**Table 1**).[8] They tend to have poor bony and cartilaginous framework with tips that have a tendency for poor rotation and projection. Nostrils can have a tendency for flaring and the skin–soft tissue envelope (S-STE) can be thick (**Fig. 1**).

THE CONSULTATION

Important points need to be covered during the consultation before surgery.

Ethnic/Racial Variations

Mestizo patients today are considered mixed-race patients. Sometimes, knowing where patients come from can help define racial characteristics, which can help to plan a surgery.

Patient's Desires/What Is Considered Beautiful by the Patient

This, for the author, is the most important part of the consultation. We need to listen to our patients and clearly understand what they want and what they consider beautiful. It is not surprising to have a patient tell you they want a "natural-looking nose," which when computer imaging is performed results in a smaller nose with more refined-looking characteristics.

Table 1
General nasal characteristics in mestizo patients

Anatomic Structure	Characteristics
Skin type	Normal to thick/sebaceous/oily
Skin–soft tissue envelope	Thick/tendency toward inflammation
Nasal bones	Normal to short
Bony dorsum	Normal to low radix Wide nasal bridge Small pseudohump
Cartilaginous nasal vault	Normal to weak, wide
Nasal tip/alar cartilages	Flimsy/unsupportive/wide/undefined Poor tip recoil
Columella	Normal to short
Nasolabial angle	Normal to acute
Nasal spine	Normal to short
Nostril shape	Horizontal shape/sometimes flaring
Alar base	Normal to wide

Adapted from Cobo R. Ethnic rhinoplasty. HNO. 2018;66(1):6–14; with permission.

Previous Surgical and Nonsurgical Procedures on the Nose

It is imperative to ask if the patient has had any surgical procedures performed including functional procedures. In Latin American countries, septoplasties are usually combined with cosmetic procedures and it is not uncommon to find patients with sequelae of previous rhinoplasties saying they only had a septoplasty performed.

Additionally, today it has become crucial to ask patients if they have had any injections on their noses. The use of injectables (nonsurgical rhinoplasty) is becoming

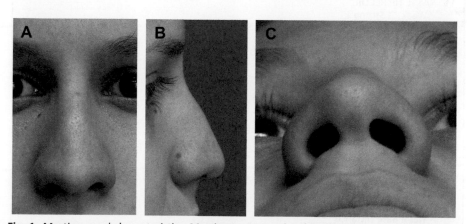

Fig. 1. Mestizo nasal characteristics. Mestizo noses tend to be mesorrhine noses. Skin has a tendency to be thick. Bony and cartilaginous framework tends to be poor. In the frontal view (*A*), the skin is thick, and nasal tips look bulbous and undefined. It is not uncommon to find small humps or pseudohumps on the lateral views (*B*) with nasal tips with poor projection and rotation. On the base view (*C*), the columella is short and the ala thick and flaring. Tips can show poor support and definition.

Table 2
Nasal evaluation chart

1. SKIN TYPE:
   Normal ☐ Thick ☐ Thin ☐ Sebaceous ☐ Dry ☐ Acne ☐
2. NASAL VALVE: N:normal C:compromised
   Internal Nasal Valve: Right☐ Left ☐
   External Nasal Valve: Right☐ Left ☐
3. NASAL SEPTUM
   Straight ☐
   Deviated: Right ☐ Left ☐
   Area of Cottle (1-4):
   Caudal ☐ Basal _____ Cephalic _____
4. INFERIOR TURBINATES
   Normal ☐ Augmented ☐ Other_____
5. NASAL BONY DORSUM
   Height of Radix in mm:_____
   Normal ☐ Low ☐ High ☐ Hump ☐ Narrow ☐ Wide ☐
   Deviated: Right ☐ Left ☐
   Depression: Right ☐ Left ☐
6. UPPER LATERAL CARTILAGES
   Normal ☐ Wide ☐ Narrow ☐
   Collapse: Right ☐ Left ☐
   Deformity:_____
7. NASAL TIP
   Alar Cartilages: Normal ☐ Thin ☐ Wide ☐ Strong ☐ Flimsy☐ Scar Tissue ☐
   Pinched: Right ☐ Left ☐
   Other: _____
8. NASOLABIAL ANGLE
   Degrees:_____ Acute☐ Obtuse ☐
9. NASAL BASE
   Normal ☐ Narrow ☐ Wide ☐ Asymmetric ☐
10. NOSTRIL ORIENTATION
    Oval ☐ Vertical ☐ Horizontal ☐
    Flaring ☐ Non-Flaring ☐
11. NASAL TIP RECOIL
    Weak ☐ Strong ☐
    Nasal Spine: Normal ☐ Prominent ☐ Small ☐ Deviated: ☐ _____
12. DONOR SITES FOR CARTILAGE GRAFTS
    Nasal Septum ☐ Auricle: Right ☐ Left ☐ Rib ☐
13. NASAL DEVIATION
    Straight: ☐
    Deviated: ☐
       Upper Third: Right ☐ Left ☐
       Middle Third: Right ☐ Left ☐
       Lower Third (Nasal Tip): Right ☐ Left: ☐
14. MEASUREMENTS (mm)
    N-T: _____
    A-T: _____
    Height of Radix_____
    Height of Rhinion_____
    Intercanthal Distance_____
    Nasal Base Distance_____

increasingly popular and it is not uncommon to find patients with permanent inject-ables in their nose. Methylmethacrylate, paraffin, and other non–Food and Drug Administration accepted permanent fillers are used frequently in nonsurgical proced-ures. Patients need to understand that it is virtually impossible to resect all of this material and that depending on where it has been injected it can seriously compromise vascularity of the nasal skin.

Physical Examination/Anatomic Diagnosis/Definition of Problems

A precise physical examination must always be performed where functional and cosmetic aspects of the nose should be documented including evaluation of the internal and external nasal valves, septum, and turbinates. A thorough checklist detailing the important aspects of the physical examination is shown in **Table 2**.

Photo Documentation/Digital Imaging

Standard rhinoplasty photographs are always taken and used to perform digital imaging analysis with the patient. Morphing of images has become a must in rhinoplasty surgery for the author. This exercise helps the patient see realistic images of what can be obtained in surgery and it also helps the surgeon define what exactly are the patient's expectations.

Definition of Surgical Options

Latin American patients frequently want noses that look smaller and more refined. This is a challenge especially when faced with noses that have a poor bony and cartilaginous structure. In the author's hands surgery is usually oriented toward reinforcing support structures and creating definition without creating noses that have too much bulk or look too big.

Discussion of Complications and Limitations of the Procedure

It is important for patients to understand that rhinoplasty is not an easy operation. Results are never perfect. The aim is to improve form and function and ideally have a patient that is happy with his or her result. All complications and limitations should be discussed openly and patients should have the opportunity to ask all the pertinent questions about their surgery. Written recommendations are given to the patient and consent forms are routinely signed.

STRUCTURAL APPROACH TO THE MESTIZO/LATINO/HISPANIC NOSE

The author has used a structural approach when performing rhinoplasty in mestizo patients for more than 20 years. The philosophy behind this approach is as follows:

- Conservative or no tissue excision
- Preservation and reinforcement of nasal support structures

Table 3
Problem solving in the upper and middle third of the nose

Problem	Surgical Solution
Upper third of nose	
Wide dorsum no hump	Medial and lateral osteotomies
Low radix/small pseudohump	Radix graft/hump remodeling with rasps
Low dorsum	Dorsal augmentation with diced cartilage plus fibrin glue and fascia
Middle third of nose	
Weak upper lateral cartilages	Spreader grafts/spreader flaps Mattress flaring sutures Onlay grafts

- Structural grafting to reinforce and increase strength of existing anatomic structures
- Cartilage remodeling with suturing techniques

To help plan surgery in a proper and efficient manner, the nose is divided into anatomic thirds as follows:

- Upper third: bony nasal dorsum
- Middle third: cartilaginous dorsum (upper lateral cartilages)
- Lower third: nasal tip (pedestal/alar cartilages/nasal base)

The upper and middle third of the nose is usually dealt with (including osteotomies) before final tip procedures are done. Surgical solutions are multiple and are usually defined depending on the problem that needs solving (**Tables 3** and **4**).[9–11]

PROBLEM SOLVING IN MESTIZO RHINOPLASTY

Structural support is the main problem with mestizo patients. It becomes crucial to harvest cartilage in a wise manner leaving a strong inverted L of cartilage of at least 10 to 15 mm dorsally and caudally. It Is not only how much septal cartilage is harvested but also how much is left behind. When cutting the septal cartilage, cutting lines should be curved and not done at sharp angles especially in the portion of the caudal and dorsal portion, the keystone area, and inferiorly in the posterior septal angle (**Fig. 2**).[12] The next decision that needs to be made is: Where am I going to

Table 4	
Problem solving in the lower third of the nose	
Problem	**Surgical Solution**
The nasal pedestal	
Retrusive/weak caudal septum	Septal extension graft
Normal caudal septum	Columellar strut
The alar cartilages	
Wide alar cartilages	Cephalic trim of lateral crura Lateral crura turn-in-flap
Long alar cartilages	Lateral crura overlay/medial crura overlay
Undefined domes/dome in abnormal position	Dome-defining suture/lateral crural steal/posterior domal sutures
Weak lateral crura of alar cartilages	Lateral crural strut graft/batten grafts
Malpositioning of alar cartilages	Angled dome-defining sutures Lateral crural repositioning
The nasal base	
Wide nasal base with flaring nostrils	Alar base/sill reduction
Weak lateral sidewall	
Weak lateral crura Malpositioned alar cartilage	Alar rim grafts Articulated alar rim grafts Lateral crural repositioning
Poor definition	
Poor definition of nasal tip	Superiorly pediculated superficial musculoaponeurotic system flap Finely diced cartilage over nasal tip Cartilage paste over nasal tip

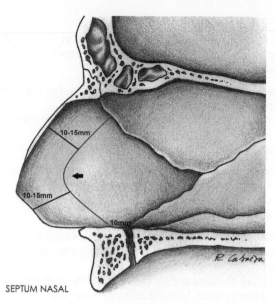

Fig. 2. Harvesting of septal cartilage. Septal cartilage should be harvested making curved incision lines especially at the keystone area (*red line*), at the junction of the caudal edge and the dorsal edge (*black arrow*), and inferiorly at the posterior septal angle preserving at least 10-mm width of cartilage inferiorly in this area.

use the cartilage I grafted? What type of grafts will be used? What are the patient's needs?

It is out of the scope of this article to describe all possible techniques that could be used when performing rhinoplasty in these patients. The author focuses in mentioning important tips on the decision-making process and how specific problems are approached today.

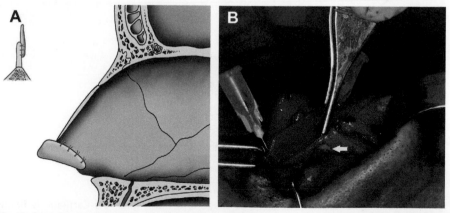

Fig. 3. Septal extension graft. (*A*) The septal extension graft is usually carved from a straight piece of cartilage and is usually placed overlapping the existing edge of the caudal septum. (*B*) Shape and position of the graft is tailored to patients' needs depending on amount of rotation and projection required. Septal extension graft sutured in place (*black arrow*). Existing caudal edge of septum (*yellow arrow*).

The Nasal Skeleton

The backbone of rhinoplasty in the author's hands is structuring the nasal skeleton before performing any tip work. This skeleton includes performing work on structuring the nasal pedestal. Two tips must be kept in mind:

- If the middle third of the nose is going to be dissected open, it should be structured with spreader flaps and/or spreader grafts
- The caudal septum should be meticulously fixed in the midline

The Nasal Pedestal

The author considers the nasal pedestal as an important support for the nasal tip. Even though the columellar strut has traditionally been used to give support to the nasal tip, when the caudal septum is retrusive or small (common in mestizo patients), it is common to use septal extension grafts (SEG) (**Fig. 3**).

- The indications for SEG are: severely acute nasolabial angles, retrusive or weak caudal septums, retrusive columellas with heavy alas, or any patient needing significant support on the nasal tip.[9]
- A straight piece of cartilage should be used for the graft and it is tailored depending on the patient's needs. In most primary rhinoplasty cases septal cartilage is used for the SEG. In mestizo patients it is not infrequent to find that it is not thick so an end-to-side (overlapping) SEG is used mostly by the author.
- The shape of the SEG is tailored depending on the patient's needs (rotation/counterrotation/projection) and its position over the caudal end of the septum varies.

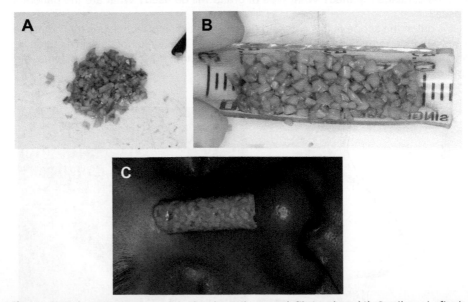

Fig. 4. Dorsal augmentation with diced cartilage and fibrin glue. (*A*) Cartilage is finely diced. (*B*) Diced cartilage is placed in template made with a 3-mL syringe cut in half and opened like a canoe. Cartilage pieces are mixed with fibrin glue and shaped according to patient's needs. (*C*) Cartilage graft placed over patient's dorsum to measure length. The dorsal portion of the graft is covered with temporalis fascia or perichondrium to avoid visible irregularities on the dorsum.

- The overlapping portion of the graft is thinned at the nasal valve area to avoid postsurgical nasal obstruction.
- Nasal tip position is defined and feet of the medial crura are stabilized to the "new" caudal septum using the tongue-in-groove technique.[13]

The Upper and Middle Third of the Nose

Mestizo patients do not usually have big noses with important osteocartilaginous humps. The problem with our patients is usually the poor structural framework that results in small humps or pseudohumps and small nasal bones with weak upper lateral cartilages.

- Bony reduction is usually conservative and performed mainly with rasps.
- If any work is going to be done in the middle third of the nose the area is strengthened with spreader flaps and/or spreader grafts.
- All cartilage in the middle third of the nose is preserved and used as autografts.
- Currently the author does not use implants for dorsal augmentation.
- All dorsal augmentation is performed using diced cartilage with fibrin glue. The dorsal portion of the graft is covered with perichondrium or temporalis fascia to avoid any visible irregularities on the dorsum over time. The author has been using this technique for more than 5 years with excellent follow-up results (**Fig. 4**). If septal cartilage is not enough, ear cartilage is harvested with good results.

The Nasal Tip

Mestizo nasal tips are a challenge to the rhinoplasty surgeon. Patients usually want nasal tips with greater definition, more refined looking but not necessarily bigger. This becomes a challenge. To be able to create definition means using grafts and

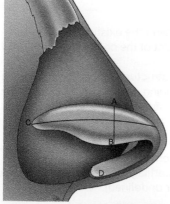
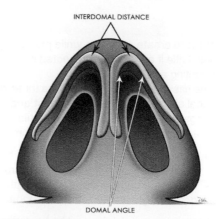
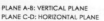

PLANE A-B: VERTICAL PLANE
PLANE C-D: HORIZONTAL PLANE

Fig. 5. Components of alar cartilages. (*Left*) Image depicts the vertical and horizontal plane. Plane A-B is the vertical component, which defines how wide the alar cartilage is and defines its concavity or convexity. Plane C-D is the horizontal component and defines length of alar cartilage. (*Right*) Image shows the horizontal component of both alar cartilages. It becomes important to define the domal angle, the interdomal distance, and the characteristics of the alar cartilages as a whole.

Table 5
Gradual approach to the nasal tip

Anatomic Finding	Surgical Solution
Management of the vertical component	
Suturing techniques	
Wide alar cartilage	Cephalic trim of medial portion of lateral crura Lateral crural turn in flap
Grafts on the nasal tip	
Concave or convex lateral crura of alar cartilages	Lateral crural strut graft Alar batten grafts
Management of the horizontal component	
Suturing techniques	
Underprojection/ underrotation of nasal tip	Lateral crural steal Dome-defining sutures Posterior domal suture Intercrural suture Septocolumellar suture
Increased interdomal distance	Lateral crural spanning sutures Alar crural spanning suture Incomplete strip procedures (cartilage dividing techniques)
Overprojected tip/long plunging nose	Lateral crural overlay technique Medial crural overlay technique
Grafts on the nasal tip	
Bulbous undefined nasal tip	Shield graft
Buckling or flaring of lateral alar sidewalls	Alar rim grafts Articulated alar rim grafts
Cephalic malposition, pinched nasal tip	Lateral crural repositioning

sutures to create structure while preserving or remodeling the existing nasal tip cartilages. Little if any tissue is resected in the nasal tip. Most of the changes are obtained reorienting and structuring.[9,10]

The nasal tip should be seen as a three-dimensional structure. Alar cartilages have a vertical and a horizontal component and surgical planning is done depending on the findings at this level (**Fig. 5**). Alar cartilages are paired structures, so the left and right cartilage should be compared for symmetry.

- Vertical component (A-B): width of the cartilage/is the shape concave or convex. Does it have a favorable or unfavorable orientation?
- Horizontal component (C-D): length of the alar cartilage. Characteristics of the domal angle (acute, obtuse, pinched, defined, or undefined).

A gradual approach is used by the author in all mestizo tips starting from more simple and predictable procedures and reserving the more aggressive unpredictable techniques for those tips that need more modifications. Sutures and grafts are used to modify these structures and little resection is performed keeping in mind the structural approach (**Table 5**).[9,14,15] For more than 5 years the author has stopped using nonabsorbable sutures on the nasal tip and uses absorbable material exclusively (5–0 polydioxanone suture).

Refining Techniques on the Nose

Camouflaging techniques are routinely used by the author to help hide irregularities, improve definition, or correct asymmetries. For many years the author routinely used morselized cartilage to cover the nasal tip area. Today and for the past 2 years we have been using finely diced cartilage and/or cartilage paste with good consistent results.[16,17]

The finely diced cartilage or paste is injected at the end of the surgery either with a cartilage injector or with a 1-mL tuberculin syringe. Its uses are multiple. It is used to fill in concavities; smooth out irregularities; augment small areas, such as the radix or supratip area; and is used to increase refinement in the nasal tip area over the domes.

Management of the Skin–Soft Tissue Envelope

Evaluation and management of the S-STE in mestizo patients is a must because their skin tends to be thicker, oilier, and with a tendency to develop acne. Elasticity of the

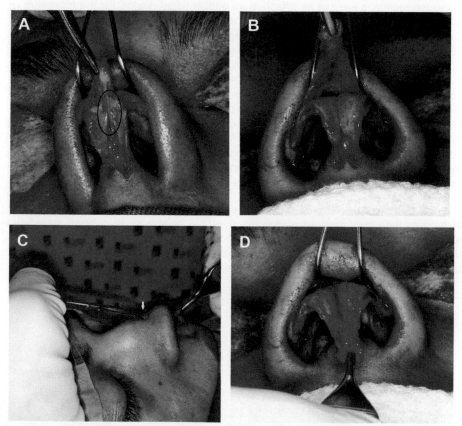

Fig. 6. Superiorly pediculated SMAS ligament flap. This is a flap with a superiorly created pedicle that eliminates dead space in the supratip area, helps accentuate the supratip break, and serves as an additional covering of tissue over the nasal tip. (*A*) SMAS flap elevated en bloc with ligament structures of the nasal tip. *Black oval* signals Pitanguy ligament, which will be elevated en bloc with SMAS. (*B*) SMAS ligament flap elevated up to supratip region where pedicle is attached. (*C*) When SMAS ligament flap is pulled down, the supratip break is marked (*yellow arrow*), which is the superiorly based pedicle of the flap. (*D*) SMAS ligament flap is lowered at the end of surgery covering all nasal tip work that was performed including sutures and grafts.

skin is reduced and it is not infrequent to find that inflammatory response is augmented resulting postsurgically in more edema of the nasal tip. The S-STE is treated medically and surgically.

Medical treatment of the skin–soft tissue envelope

Skin thickness is classified in all patients and a skin regime is defined depending on the patient's individual needs. The objective of treatment is to re-establish the patient's normal skin condition and to reduce inflammatory response as much as possible. Skin programs are targeted toward cleansing, exfoliation, and control of oil and sebum production.[18]

In skin type III patients or patients with thick acne-prone oily skin, in addition to topical treatments, low-dose oral isotretinoin (13-cis-retinoic acid) is recommended.[19] Patients are started on a low-dose treatment (0.025–0.40 mg/kg/d) unless a higher dose is recommended because of severe acne. Recent studies have shown that low-dose regimens are just as effective as conventional dosing for the treatment of acne, the medication is better tolerated, the side effects are less, and there is no increase in relapse of acne. Treatment regimens are continued for approximately 16 weeks until the skin is completely cleared.

In patients who are already on isotretinoin before surgery, the medication is stopped 1 week before the procedure and restarted after tapes are taken off the skin (10–15 days after surgery). Today, no evidence supports delaying skin surgery, or using dermabrasion or superficial chemical peels.[20,21] Patients who have not started isotretinoin before surgery safely start their low-dose regimens 2 weeks after the surgical procedure when nasal tapes have come off. All patients who are taking oral isotretinoin should be monitored closely with laboratory tests that include hepatic function tests and pregnancy tests. Pregnancy is an absolute contraindication for isotretinoin use and contraceptive measures should be taken by men and women alike.

Surgical treatment of the skin–soft tissue envelope

In patients with thick inelastic skin sometimes it is necessary to perform superficial musculoaponeurotic system (SMAS) debulking or resection over the supratip and tip area taking care to respect the subdermal plexus. If this is done in a conservative fashion, without using cautery or being aggressive with its resection, it can help create

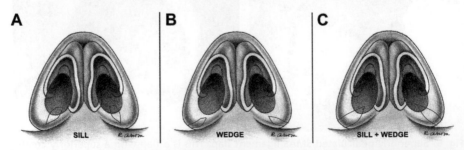

Fig. 7. Alar base resection. Three basic techniques are used when performing alar base resection. (*A*) Alar sill resection is used in patients who have a wide nasal base with little or no alar flaring. Incision is extended into nasal sill without a lateral extension into the ala. (*B*) Alar wedge resection is used in patients who have important alar flaring with normal sills. Incision is extended laterally following alar crease. After meticulous closure, ala is shortened and flare reduced. (*C*) Nostril sill and alar wedge resection is used when alar base is wide and has excessive flaring. After meticulous closure, ala is shortened, flare reduced, and interalar distance diminished.

definition over the nasal tip area, although it is not a surgical maneuver that is performed routinely.

Elimination of dead space over the supratip area is important to help reduce inflammation and to prevent scar tissue formation in this area. When elevating the skin flap of the external approach, the author routinely dissects a superiorly pediculated SMAS ligament flap. At the end of surgery after all tip work has been done the flap is lowered and sutured back in place covering all nasal tip work. The use of the flap is two-fold: it

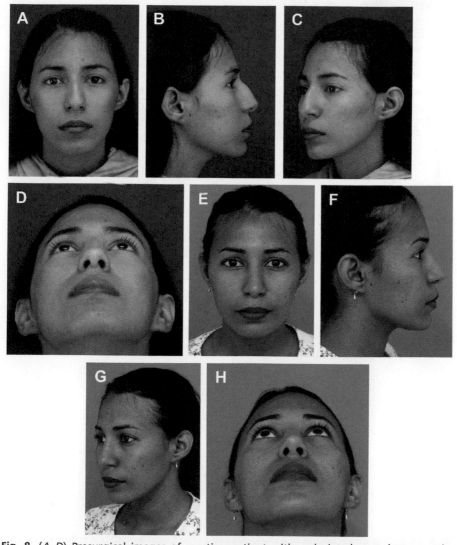

Fig. 8. (*A–D*) Presurgical images of mestizo patient with a deviated nose; hump; and a bulbous, underprojected, and asymmetric nasal tip. (*E–H*) Three-year postsurgical images after hump reduction, medial and lateral osteotomies, spreader grafts, and spreader flaps. The nasal tip projection was increased with the placement of a septal extension graft and tip-defining sutures. Refinement techniques with finely diced cartilage and cartilage paste were used in the radix, the rhinion, and the nasal tip. A superiorly pediculated SMAS ligament flap was used to help camouflage any possible nasal tip irregularities.

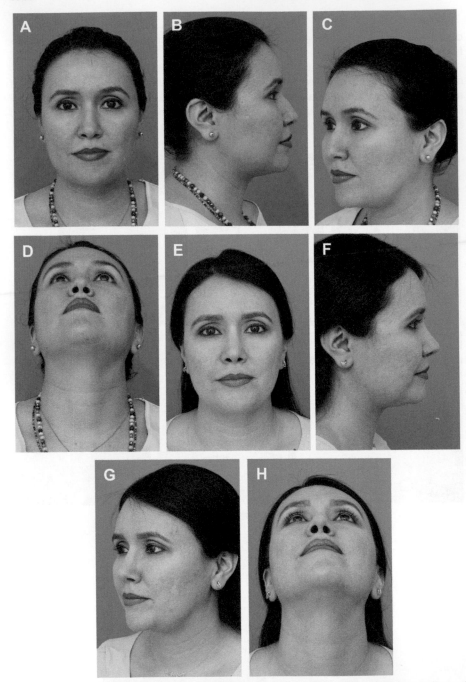

Fig. 9. (*A–D*) Presurgical images of a thick-skinned patient with a small hump; low radix; and underprojected, rounded nasal tip. (*E–H*) Two-year postsurgical images after conservative hump removal, placement of spreader grafts and spreader flaps, and medial and lateral osteotomies. Nasal tip projection was obtained with a strong septal extension graft and tip-defining sutures. Finely diced cartilage and cartilage paste were placed in the radix, the rhinion, and the nasal tip. A superiorly pediculated SMAS ligament flap was used as a covering over the nasal tip. Patient's thick skin was treated postsurgically during 6 months with a low-dose scheme of oral isotretinoin twice a week.

decreases the dead space over the supratip area and serves as a covering of all grafts that have been placed over the nasal tip. Once the flap is sutured in place, finely diced cartilage or cartilage paste is injected over the dome area or alar cartilages to give additional refinement or camouflage to the nasal tip. The SMAS covering helps keep the paste or the finely diced cartilage pieces in place (**Fig. 6**).[22]

The Nasal Base

Alar base reduction is not a standard procedure in mestizo patients. It is not uncommon to find that after all surgical techniques have been performed the nasal base has changed, the alar flaring has been corrected, and there is no need to perform procedures in the nasal base.

Three basic techniques are used when performing surgery on the nasal base (**Fig. 7**):

- Nostril sill excision: This is used for wide nasal base with little or no flaring.
- Alar wedge excision: This shortens the ala and corrects the alar flare. It does not correct a wide nasal base and the incision does not enter the nostril.
- Nostril sill plus alar wedge excision: This is used when the alar base is wide and there is excessive flaring.

Postsurgical Follow-up

Close follow-up is a necessity in mestizo patients because of their S-STE characteristics. Stitches are removed on Day 5 to 7 with the cast, and additional taping of the nose is done for an extra week. Excessive use of taping on the nose is not encouraged because this promotes sebum formation and exacerbates oiliness.

Topical skin regimes are started as soon as tapes come off. When patients need oral isotretinoin (discussed previously), this is also started 2 weeks after surgery when tapes come off. It is important to emphasize that sun exposure should be avoided the first months because this worsens dark circles under the eyes and increases nasal edema. The same thing goes for active exercise, such as running and kickboxing, which should be avoided during the first months after surgery.

In general, patients should be able to resume their normal daily activities after 2 weeks with the limitations mentioned previously. Follow-up visits are scheduled at 3 months, 6 months, 9 months, 1 year, and 18 months. Pictures are taken at 6 months, 9 months, 1 year, and 18 months. After the first 18 months patients are encouraged to come in on a yearly basis (**Figs. 8** and **9**).

SUMMARY

Rhinoplasty is the number one facial plastic surgical procedure performed in mestizo, Latino, or Hispanic patients. Mestizo, or mixed race, patients comprise the biggest minority group in the United States. Mestizo noses are mesorrhine noses that have a tendency to have poor osteocartilaginous framework with a thicker S-STE.

When performing rhinoplasty, it becomes imperative to clearly define what the patient wants before performing any surgical procedure. A structural approach has been used for many years where techniques are focused on anatomic findings and on reinforcing support structures of the nose while creating better definition and refinement of nasal structures and resecting little if any tissue of the nose. The final ideal result should be a balanced-looking nose that blends in with the patient's face and can withstand the natural healing process. Preservation of ethnic features is not as important as giving patients results that bring them closer to their aesthetic ideal.

DISCLOSURE

The author has nothing to disclose.

REFERENCES

1. Available at: https://www.merriam-webster.com/dictionary/mestizo. Accessed August 9, 2019.
2. Available at: https://www.pewresearch.org/fact-tank/2015/07/10/mestizo-and-mulatto-mixed-race-identities-unique-to-hispanics/. Accessed August 9, 2019.
3. Available at: https://www.britannica.com/story/whats-the-difference-between-hispanic-and-latino. Accessed August 9, 2019.
4. Available at: https://www.census.gov/topics/population/hispanic-origin/about.html. Accessed August 9, 2019.
5. Daniel RK. Hispanic rhinoplasty in the United States, with emphasis on the Mexican American nose. Plast Reconstr Surg 2003;112:244–56 [discussion: 257–8].
6. Ortiz-Monasterio F, Olmedo A. Rhinoplasty on the mestizo nose. Clin Plast Surg 1977;4:89–102.
7. Milgrim L, Lawson W, Cohen AF. Anthropometric analysis of the female Latino nose. Arch Otolaryngol Head Neck Surg 1996;122:1079–86.
8. Cobo R. Ethnic rhinoplasty. HNO 2018;66(1):6–14.
9. Cobo R. Rhinoplasty in Latino patients. Clin Plast Surg 2016;43:237–54.
10. Cobo R. Hispanic/mestizo rhinoplasty. Facial Plast Surg Clin North Am 2010; 18(1):173–88.
11. Cobo R. Rhinoplasty in the mestizo nose. Facial Plast Surg Clin North Am 2014; 22(3):395–415.
12. Jeong JY. Obtaining maximal stability with a septal extension technique in East Asian rhinoplasty. Arch Plast Surg 2014;41:19–28.
13. Kridel RW, Scott BA, Foda HM. The tongue-in-groove technique in septorhinoplasty. A 10 year experience. Arch Facial Plast Surg 1999;1:246–56.
14. Toriumi D, Asher S. Lateral crural repositioning for treatment of cephalic malposition. Facial Plast Surg Clin North Am 2015;23:55–71.
15. Goodrich JL, Wong BJF. Optimizing the soft tissue triangle, alar margin furrow, and alar ridge aesthetics: analysis and use of the articulate alar rim graft. Facial Plast Surg 2016;32:646–55.
16. Kreutzer C, Hoehne J, Gubisch W, et al. Free diced cartilage. Plast Reconstr Surg 2017;140(3):461–70.
17. Erol OO. Injection of compressed diced cartilage in the correction of secondary and primary rhinoplasty. Plast Reconstr Surg 2017;140(5):673e–85e.
18. Cobo R, Camacho JG, Orrego J. Integrated management of the thick-skinned rhinoplasty patient. Facial Plast Surg 2018;34:3–8.
19. Cobo R, Vitery L. Isotretinoin use in thick-skinned rhinoplasty patients. Facial Plast Surg 2016;32(06):656–61.
20. Spring LK, Krakowski AC, Alam M, et al. Isotretinoin and timing of procedural interventions: a systematic review with consensus recommendations. JAMA Dermatol 2017;153(08):802–9.
21. Zaenglein AL, Pathy AL, Schlosser BJ, et al. Guidelines of care for the management of acne vulgaris. J Am Acad Dermatol 2016;74(05):945–73.e33.
22. Cobo R. Superiorly pediculated musculoaponeurotic system ligament flap to control the supratip. JAMA Facial Plast Surg 2018;20(6):513–4.

Surgical Considerations in Patients of Middle Eastern Descent

Robert Deeb, MD

KEYWORDS

- Middle Eastern rhinoplasty • Ethnic rhinoplasty • Nasal surgery
- Cosmetic rhinoplasty

KEY POINTS

- Rhinoplasty in Middle Eastern patients presents a unique challenge given the heterogeneity in patient skin tone and thickness, nasal structure, and surgical goals.
- Nasofacial analysis and photography play a particularly important role given the often disparate views the patient may hold of their nasal deformity relative to the surgeon.
- Honest and candid conversations regarding goals and realistic expectations are required.
- Goals of the surgery are a natural-appearing nose with adequate support and preservation of nasal function, which are usually achieved by conservative, structure-preserving maneuvers.

INTRODUCTION

The Middle East is a region encompassing southwest Asia and northern Africa, encompassing more than 20 countries. It is an ethnically diverse area with many languages and cultures. Although definitions may vary, a more inclusive interpretation of the region comprises the countries of northern Africa, the Arabian Peninsula, the Levant, Turkey, and Iran.[1]

Rhinoplasty in patients of Middle Eastern descent presents a unique challenge for a variety of reasons. There is a tremendous amount of heterogeneity in facial features with all eye colors, skin tones, and facial structures being represented. Although some patterns exist in the types of patients who seek rhinoplasty, there needs to be an individualized approach to surgical planning and patient care. Emphasis should be placed on performing conservative maneuvers to achieve a balanced, natural-appearing nose that preserves the patient's ethnic heritage.

Division of Facial Plastic and Reconstructive Surgery, Department of Otolaryngology–Head and Neck Surgery, Henry Ford Health System, Henry Ford Hospital, 2799 West Grand Boulevard, Detroit, MI 48202, USA
E-mail address: rdeeb1@hfhs.org

Otolaryngol Clin N Am 53 (2020) 283–298
https://doi.org/10.1016/j.otc.2019.11.001
0030-6665/20/© 2019 Elsevier Inc. All rights reserved.

PREOPERATIVE CONSULTATION
Patient Attitudes and Goals

Although the office consultation holds significant importance in all rhinoplasty patients, it is especially critical in the Middle Eastern patient. The patient tends to hold a certain view of their nose, which can be quite different from that of the surgeon. It is a mistake to view this group of patients as monolithic. Patients often have varying goals and expectations. It is important to delve into the patient's specific reason for pursuing surgery and what exact changes they are hoping to achieve.

A religiously appropriate greeting should be respected, as often women are not permitted to shake hands with a man, who is a nonfamily member. It is not uncommon for an adult female patient to be accompanied by her father, husband, or brother. Patients of the Islamic faith may wear a head scarf (hijab), which may obstruct some facial features. These may need to be fully or partially removed to fully examine the nose and face. Obviously, permission should be granted before undertaking the physical examination.

It is essential to get a sense of the patient's grasp of the English language. If the patient speaks English poorly, the importance of a translator cannot be overstated. Although there may be a family member present who speaks English more proficiently than the patient, this person should not be used as the translator. A trained, professional with experience in medical translation should be used whenever possible.

There are also culturally sensitive discussions regarding the patient's desire to maintain certain aspects of their ethnicity while wanting to modify others. The patient's immigration history may be important because it often affects their view of their ethnicity. Recent immigrants to the United States are often more likely to want to maintain many of their traditional features, whereas American-born patients of Middle Eastern descent may have a desire for a more westernized nose.[2]

It is critical to assess for any underlying psychiatric disease, specifically body dysmorphic disorder.[3] A patient's desire to achieve an unnatural appearing nose or the nose of a different person is a warning sign that should not be ignored.

Expectations and Functional Concerns

Nasal surgery in the Middle East is quite common.[4] The Rhinology Research Society of Iran conducted a study in cooperation with Johns Hopkins University and found that the rate of rhinoplasty in Iran per capita is seven times that of America.[5] In addition, it is often performed by a variety of practitioners with varying levels of expertise and training. In fact, in Tehran, Iran, there are only 157 licensed plastic surgeons but there are 7000 unlicensed surgeons.[5]

As such, one must take a detailed history of the types of previous procedures that have been performed. If any of these procedures have led to any improvement or worsening of symptoms, it should be noted. Timing of the procedures as well as whether or not any allografts or autografts have been placed must be ascertained.

If the patient is experiencing functional deficits in addition to their cosmetic concerns, those issues require special attention during the consultation. It is important to establish if the patient is being driven by cosmetic concerns, functional concerns, or both. Standardized, validated quality of life instruments such as the Nasal Obstruction Symptom Evaluation (NOSE) scale can be useful in this regard.[6] The NOSE scale is a brief, valid, reliable, and responsive survey to measure disturbances in the quality of life specific to nasal obstruction.[7] A thorough history and physical examination investigating all possible causes of the patient's symptoms is of paramount importance. Specific attention to allergic symptoms as well as the cardinal symptoms of chronic sinusitis should be pursued as well.[8] Nasal endoscopy as well as possible use of computed tomography (if sinus disease is suspected) is encouraged. Assessment of the internal and external nasal valves should be done as part of routine physical examination.

Photography

Standardized photography of the patient in frontal view, basal view, and bilateral oblique and lateral views should be obtained during the preoperative consultation. These photos should be taken with the patient in the repose as well as during animation with natural smiling. Patients will sometimes bring photos of themselves to highlight their cosmetic concerns. Care should be taken to assess these photos with a wary eye, especially if taken as a "selfie." A recent study by Ward and colleagues[9] showed that short-distance photography increases the perceived ratio of nasal breadth to bizygomatic breadth, which has the net effect of making the nose look larger. Whenever possible, use standardized, clinical photos to discuss the patient's concerns as well as any possible goals and expectations.

Patients may bring images of their nose that they have altered using commercially available software applications. Although these can be helpful to ascertain the patient's goals, it is essential to have a frank discussion regarding feasibility of certain changes. This is especially true in patients with thick skin who desire dramatic narrowing of the dorsum or nasal tip.

In addition, the surgeon may choose to use digital image modification software to aid in the preoperative discussion of possible outcomes. Again, this should be used with caution as to not give the patient unrealistic expectations. Punthakee and colleagues[10] showed that ratings by patients and surgeons comparing preoperative modified images with postoperative outcomes is predictive in approximately 75% of patients and that lateral images are more useful for this goal. Although the digitally altered photos can act as an education tool, they should not be used to "guarantee" results.

NASOFACIAL ANALYSIS

Although there is significant heterogeneity of the nasofacial structure in patients of Middle Eastern descent, several distinctive features tend to exist in those patients seeking cosmetic rhinoplasty (**Fig. 1**). The upper two-thirds of the nose tend to be overprojected, often with a convex dorsum. A combined bony and cartilaginous dorsal hump is common although it varies in degree.

The position of the nasal tip tends to be dependent and sometimes ptotic. Tip ptosis refers to the fact that the tip is underrotated with a nasolabial angle less than 90°. Tip dependence refers to the relationship of the tip-defining point being below or ventral to the anterior septal angle, irrespective of the nasolabial angle (**Fig. 2**). As such, patients may complain of their nose looking "droopy" and yet the nasolabial angle is adequate. The combination of the ptotic and dependent nasal tip with convex dorsum gives the appearance of the pseudohump in the lateral view.[11] Nasal length is generally excessive relative to nasal tip projection.[12] On frontal view, there is often infratip lobular fullness, which may obstruct view of the upper lip (**Fig. 3**).

The lower lateral cartilages are often weak and the nasal tip tends to be underprojected. Patients nearly universally complain that their nose is "too big" or that they desire "a smaller nose"; however, tip projection, especially after dorsal reduction, is often necessary. The nasal septum tends to have relatively resilient cartilage. Autografts such as rib or ear cartilage are generally not necessary in primary rhinoplasty.

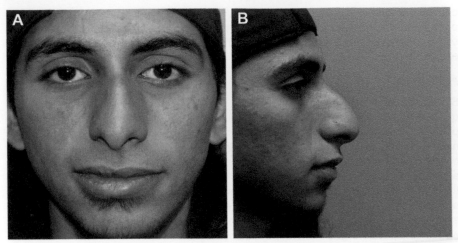

Fig. 1. Typical Middle Eastern patient seeking rhinoplasty: (*A*) frontal view and (*B*) lateral view.

Another common feature in patients of Middle Eastern descent is the smile deformity (**Fig. 4**). The smile deformity is defined by 3 components: (1) tip derotation, (2) upper lip shortening, and (3) transverse crease in the philtral area, which occurs with smiling.[13] The primary muscle acting to produce the smile deformity is the paired depressor septinasi.[14] Hyperactivity of this muscle is the likely cause of the smile deformity.[15] It is important to note that all 3 components are not necessarily present in all patients with the smile deformity. In addition, there are various degrees of severity depending on the strength of the muscle and extent of hyperactivity.

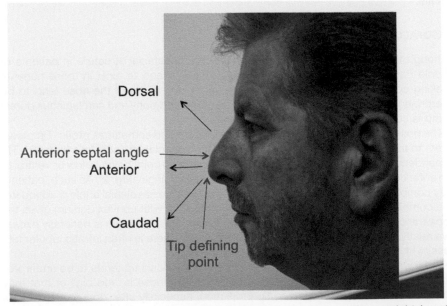

Fig. 2. Tip dependence without tip ptosis; the tip seems droopy despite a nasolabial angle greater than 90°.

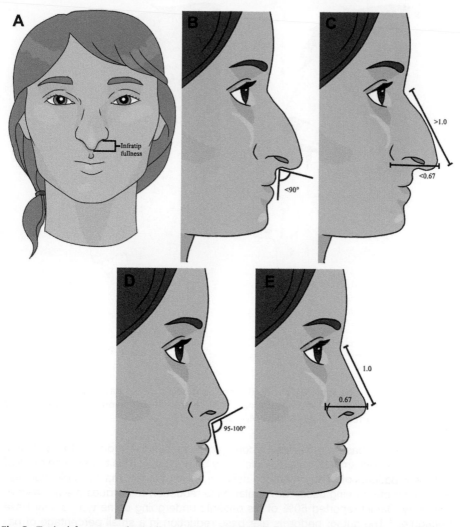

Fig. 3. Typical features of Middle Eastern nose. (*A*) Frontal view showing excessive infratip lobular fullness. (*B*) Preoperative lateral view showing inadequate nasolabial angle. (*C*) Preoperative lateral view showing dorsal convexity with increased nasal length relative to tip projection. (*D*) Postoperative lateral view showing normalized nasolabial angle. (*E*) Postoperative lateral view showing normalized ratio of nasal length to tip projection. (*Courtesy of Haley Sibley, MD, Detroit, MI.*)

The smile deformity has become a more frequently identified concern with the explosion of social media platforms in recent years.[16] Because patients have begun seeing themselves from various angles and in various lights, dynamic changes of the nose have become more apparent.

Middle Eastern patients often have thicker skin compared with Caucasian patients. This is especially true in the nasal tip where there is increased sebaceous tissue. This tends to camouflage the underlying nasal framework and often leads to an amorphous, bulbous appearance.

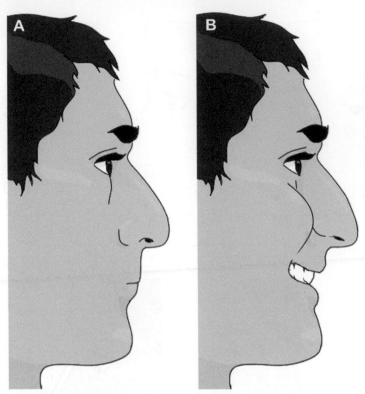

Fig. 4. Depiction of the smile deformity defined as descent of the nasal tip, shortening of the upper lip, and horizontal philtral crease. (*A*) Lateral view in repose. (*B*) Lateral view with smiling. (*Courtesy of* Haley Sibley, MD, Detroit, MI.)

Excessive alar base width is also a common complaint in Middle Eastern patients. There is a variable amount of flare, which may be present.[17] This tends to be more of an issue in patients of northern African descent. Given the fact that tip projection maneuvers are often being used, formal alar base reduction techniques are not always necessary. Daniel reported 50% of his patients undergoing some type of alar base procedure.[18] The author performs alar base reduction in a small percentage of patients. Alar base incisions should be carefully planned given the propensity for scarring associated with thicker skin types.

SURGICAL APPROACHES

Both open and closed rhinoplasty approaches are acceptable in the management of the Middle Eastern nose. The author prefers the closed approach for the usual stated benefits of avoidance of external scar, decreased tip swelling, and shorter surgical time.[19] Emphasis should be placed on conservative surgical maneuvers in hopes of achieving a balanced and natural-appearing nose. Preservation and maintenance of nasal function is of the utmost importance. Although grafting materials may be necessary, the nasal septum often acts as an adequate source in the primary rhinoplasty setting. In the case of secondary or revision rhinoplasty, additional grafting materials such as rib or auricular cartilage may be necessary.[20] Preoperative assessment of the nasal septum will help determine the amount of usable cartilage that may be necessary in the primary or secondary setting.

Management of the Nasal Dorsum

Most of the patients will require some degree of dorsal hump reduction. The dorsal hump may be entirely bony or cartilaginous, although most of them are a combination of the two. There may be a degree of asymmetry to the nasal dorsum, which requires consideration when performing reduction to ensure a balanced and symmetric result. In addition, resection of a conservative amount of the anterior septal angle is often required to treat tip dependence.

Before dorsal reduction, submucosal release of the upper lateral cartilages is often necessary to preserve a space for possible later spreader graft placement. The dorsal aspects of the upper lateral cartilages may require trimming to allow a smooth transition from the upper third of the nose to the midvault. Care should be taken to avoid overresection of the upper lateral cartilages.

Conservative reduction is essential to avoid a "scooped out" or unnatural-appearing nose on lateral view (**Fig. 5**). The amount of reduction should be discussed with the patient preoperatively, as some patients may have a desire to retain a certain amount of dorsal projection to retain their ethnic identity. Intraoperative swelling, especially in the thick-skinned patient, needs to be accounted for when setting the dorsal height. Female patients should have a slight supratip break, which is achieved with conservative reduction of the anterior septal angle as part of the dorsal reduction.

Narrowing osteotomies are nearly universally necessary following dorsal reduction to close the open roof deformity. The medial osteotomy is often achieved with the dorsal bony reduction although it can be confirmed with straight or curved osteotome. Lateral osteotomies to fully mobilize the nasal bones and allow for closure of the open roof are then necessary. If the patient has a crooked bony vault, intermediate osteotomies can be used to aid in straightening.[21] Intermediate osteotomies may also be used to manage especially wide or convex nasal bones.

Management of the Septum

Septal surgery is usually required in most cases of Middle Eastern rhinoplasty. Modifications of the nasal septum can act to relieve functional obstructions as well as aid in achieving aesthetic goals. At a minimum, it is necessary to harvest septal cartilage to use as grafting material. Emphasis should be placed on maintenance of an adequate L-strut. Only the amount of cartilage or bone necessary to achieve the desired goal should be removed. The rest should be left in situ as a possible repository in case revision surgery is necessary and to maintain nasal support.

Complex septal deviations are not uncommon. Mild caudal septal deviations can be treated with well-described maneuvers such as the swinging door technique,[22] repositioning to the midline with suture fixation, or modified Goldman technique.[23] Conservative caudal septal shave techniques can be used to improve alar-columellar disproportions such as a hanging columella. Caudal septal shave can also be used

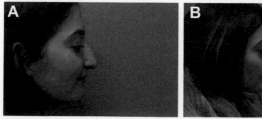

Fig. 5. Conservative dorsal reduction: (A) preoperative view and (B) postoperative view.

to aid in tip rotation maneuvers by performing an inverted triangle excision at the caudal margin.[24] However, overresection of the caudal septum should be avoided, as it may destabilize the tip or lead to loss of adequate columella show.

Severe anterocaudal septal deviations may require formal anterior septal reconstructive techniques such as full or partial extracorporeal septoplasty.[25,26] Special attention should be paid to the keystone region, as the combination of dorsal reduction and aggressive submucosal resection of the septum in this area may lead to loss of dorsal height and postoperative saddling. Maintenance of a 1-cm dorsal strut at this region is critical. Use of spreader grafts can be used to stabilize this area.

Management of the Middle Vault

Maintaining strength in the middle vault will aid in preventing postoperative complications such as nasal obstruction, inverted-V deformity, saddle nose, and pollybeak deformity. Large dorsal reductions may leave a gap in the middle vault between the dorsal septum and upper lateral cartilages despite narrowing osteotomies. In these scenarios, spreader grafting can be used to maintain dorsal strength and aid in "closing the roof" (**Fig. 6**).[27] The grafts will also act to prevent inferior displacement of the upper lateral cartilages and prevent functional issues in the postoperative setting.

Nasal Tip Surgery

Nasal tip surgery in the Middle Eastern patient requires consideration of tip position as well as nasal tip definition. Relationship of the tip-defining point to the anterior septal angle requires special attention, as reversal of tip dependence is the goal (**Fig. 7**). The nasal tip is often wide, bulbous, and amorphous. Conservative trimming of the cephalic portion of the lower lateral cartilages can aid is decreasing supratip fullness. If the lower lateral cartilages are cephalically oriented, the use of lateral crural strut grafts or alar rim grafts can aid in improving this deformity.[28,29]

As the tip tends to be ptotic and underprojected in most patients, rotation and projection maneuvers are usually used. Tip-narrowing sutures, placed in both an intradomal and interdomal fashion, are usually necessary. The author prefers to incorporate a columellar strut into the dome-binding complex in most patients (**Fig. 8**). Although the caudal septum is often strong in Middle Eastern patients, the lower lateral cartilages, specifically the medial crura, tend to be weak. A columellar strut acts to stabilize this area and provide added tip support (**Figs. 9–11**).[30]

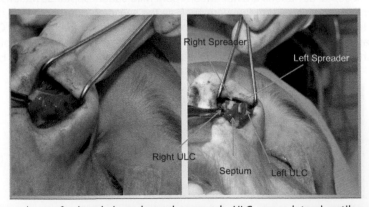

Fig. 6. Spreader graft placed via endonasal approach. ULC, upper lateral cartilage.

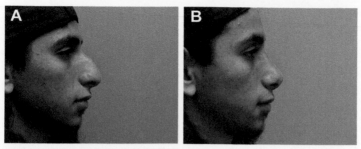

Fig. 7. Reversal of tip dependence with conservative resection of the anterior septal angle: (*A*) preoperative view and (*B*) postoperative view.

Lateral crural steal can be applied to further alter tip rotation, projection, and nasal length.[31] A recent study showed a decrease of 1.5 mm in length for each 1 mm of lateralization of the domes. The nasolabial angle increased 4.7° for every millimeter of lateralization of the domes.[32] Care should be taken not to overrotate the nasal tip, which may give an unnatural appearance. A study done in Saudi Arabia showed that the overall mean preferred nasolabial angle for men was 89.39 and the overall mean preferred angle for women was 90.62, which is somewhat less than that desired in western populations.[33] If additional tip projection is required, tip grafts may be used. Alternatively, an extended columellar strut-tip graft can be used, especially if performing endonasalrhinoplasty.[34]

Perhaps the most difficult aspect of the nasal tip to manage in the operative setting is the nasal skin. Some investigators have advocated for defatting to help improve definition and contour.[35] This should be performed with caution as to not create underlying irregularities. Tip grafting is also commonly used to aid in projection and narrowing.[36–40]

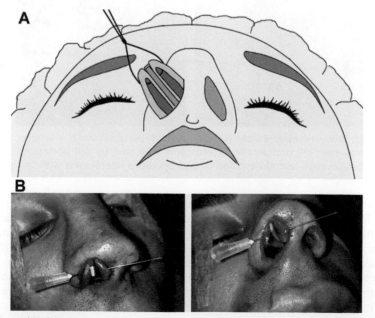

Fig. 8. Dome-binding technique incorporating columellar strut performed via an endonasal approach. (*A*) Illustration. (*B*) Photograph. ([*A*] *Courtesy of* Haley Sibley, MD, Detroit, MI.)

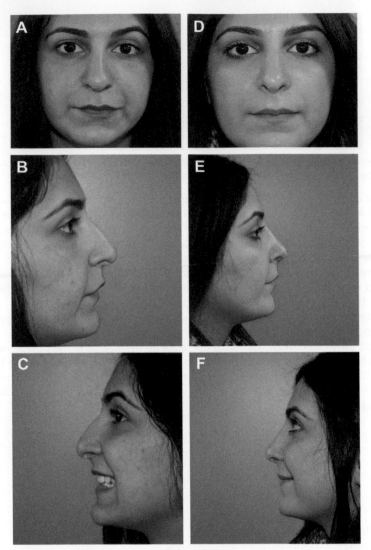

Fig. 9. Result following Middle Eastern rhinoplasty: (A) preoperative frontal view, (B) preoperative lateral view, (C) preoperative lateral view with smiling, (D) postoperative frontal view, (E) postoperative lateral view, and (F) postoperative lateral view with smiling.

The author has found alar base reduction to be unnecessary in most of the patients, as the alar base tends to decrease once the tip has been projected. In Caucasian noses, the idealized interalar distance is equivalent to the intercanthaldistance.[41] However, Middle Eastern patients are able to tolerate an increased interalar distance as well as a small amount of alar flare.[42] Alar base modification should be used as the last maneuver of the operation, following all tip maneuvers as well as osteotomies.[17] Alternatively, it may also be performed as a secondary procedure in the office setting several months or more after the primary procedure.

Treatment of the smile deformity can be accomplished in a variety of ways.[43–45] All interventions focus on alteration of the depressor septinasi muscle. The depressor

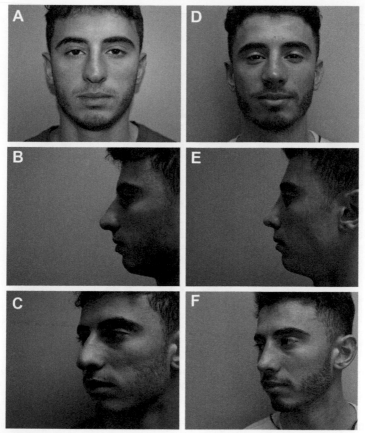

Fig. 10. Result following Middle Eastern rhinoplasty: (*A*) preoperative frontal view, (*B*) preoperative lateral view, (*C*) preoperative oblique view, (*D*) postoperative frontal view, (*E*) postoperative lateral view, and (*F*) postoperative oblique view.

septi is a paired muscle contained within the columella, which originates on the medial crura footplates and caudal septum and has variable insertion patterns in the region of the orbicularis oris and nasal spine.[15,46] The author prefers treatment of the smile deformity by extending the full transfixion incision inferiorly to the nasal spine, identifying the muscle at its attachment and excising bilaterally (**Figs. 12** and **13**).[16]

AVOIDANCE OF PITFALLS AND COMPLICATIONS

There are a variety of potential complications that can occur following rhinoplasty in the Middle Eastern patient, many of which are parallel to those of Caucasian patients.[47,48] As outlined earlier, the goals of the procedure should be a natural, aesthetically pleasing nose, with preservation of function. Avoidance of complications begins with a thorough discussion with the patient regarding their perceived deformities and concerns, as well as comprehensive nasofacial analysis.

Skin thickness is quite variable in Middle Eastern patients and should be given special consideration when selecting maneuvers. Although the rule may be that the skin tends to be thick, there are regions of the Middle East where thin, lighter skin is the

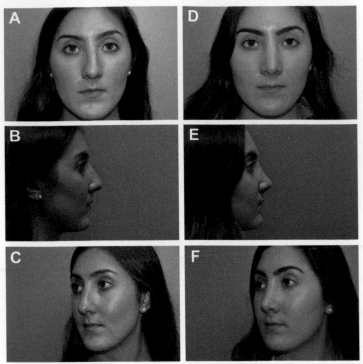

Fig. 11. Result following Middle Eastern rhinoplasty: (*A*) preoperative frontal view, (*B*) preoperative lateral view, (*C*) preoperative oblique view, (*D*) postoperative frontal view, (*E*) postoperative lateral view, and (*F*) postoperative oblique view.

norm. In patients with thinner skin, grafts should be softened and edges smoothed to avoid visible irregularities.

In order to affect change in the thick-skinned patient, more forceful techniques, such as tip grafting, lateral crural steal, and columellar strut placement are often required. These maneuvers will also help to resist tip-drop due to the heaviness of

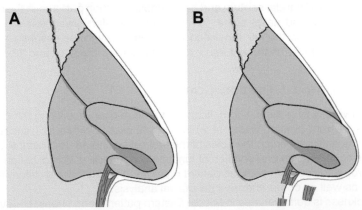

Fig. 12. (*A, B*) Resection of depressor septinasi muscle. (*Courtesy of* Haley Sibley, MD, Detroit, MI.)

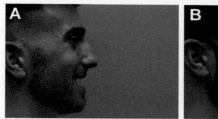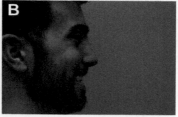

Fig. 13. Improvement in smile deformity with excision of the depressor septinasi: (A) preoperative view and (B) postoperative view.

the soft tissue skin envelope. Thick-skinned patients should be informed that postoperative swelling will persist for many months.[49] Taping has been used to help decrease edema in the postoperative setting.[50]

Overreduction of the nasal dorsum in patients with large dorsal humps should be avoided, as it can lead to the stigmata of rhinoplasty. Failure to reconstruct the keystone region after hump reduction, with or without spreader grafts, can lead to inverted-V deformity.[47] Inverted-V deformity may also result from failure to close the open roof, with narrowing osteotomies, following dorsal reduction. Saddle nose deformity may result from overly aggressive dorsal reduction.[47]

Pollybeak deformity is also a potential complication. Pollybeak deformity is defined as a convexity in the supratip region relative to the rest of the nose. There are a variety of mechanisms for this occurrence, including (1) overresection of the bony dorsum, (2) underresection of the anterior septal angle or dorsal aspects of the upper lateral cartilages, (3) loss of tip support, and (4) overresection of the anterior septal angle with resultant scar tissue filling the void.[48,51,52] In the postoperative period, pilosebaceous content of the soft tissue skin envelope can contribute to tissue scarring and pollybeak formation.[42] Nasal tip steroid shots can be used in the postoperative setting to treat asymmetric scarring and overall tip swelling.[53]

SUMMARY

Rhinoplasty in Middle Eastern patients presents a unique challenge. An individualized, patient-specific approach is required to achieve a balanced, natural result. Cultural considerations should be respected in all cases, as an overly westernized appearance is generally not desired. An honest and detail-oriented discussion is necessary as the cornerstone of the patient encounter. Preservation of function and avoidance of overly aggressive maneuvers will lead to prevention of complications and a happy patient.

ACKNOWLEDGMENT

The author would like to acknowledge and thank Haley Sibley, MD, Resident in the Department of Otolaryngology-Head and Neck Surgery at Henry Ford Hospital for her original artwork.

DISCLOSURE

The author has nothing to disclose.

REFERENCES

1. TeachMideast. What is the middle east?. Available at: http://teachmideast.org/articles/what-is-the-middle-east/. Accessed July 16, 2019.
2. Sajjadian A. Rhinoplasty in Middle Eastern patients. ClinPlastSurg 2016;43: 281–94.
3. Phillips KA. Understanding body dysmorphic disorder: an essential guide. New York: Oxford University Press; 2009.
4. KalantarMotamedi MH, Ebrahimi A, Shams A, et al. Health and social problems of rhinoplasty in Iran. World J PlastSurg 2016;5:75–6.
5. Kirkova D. Iran is the nose job capital of the world with SEVEN times more procedures than the U.S. - but rise in unlicensed surgeons poses huge risk. DailyMail.com. March 4, 2013. Available at: http://www.dailymail.co.uk/femail/article-2287961/Iran-named-nose-job-capital-world-SEVEN-times-rhinoplasty-operations-U-S-Iranian-women-strive-western-doll-face.html. Accessed July 16, 2019.
6. Stewart MG, Witsell DL, Smith TL, et al. Development and validation of the Nasal Obstruction Symptom Evaluation (NOSE) scale. OtolaryngolHeadNeckSurg 2004;130:157–63.
7. Lipan MJ, Most SP. Development of a severity classification system for subjective nasal obstruction. JAMAFacialPlastSurg 2013;15:358–61.
8. Rosenfeld RM, Andes D, Bhattacharyya N, et al. Clinical practice guideline: adult sinusitis. OtolaryngolHeadNeckSurg 2007;137:S1–31.
9. Ward B, Ward M, Fried O, et al. Nasal distortion in short-distance photographs: the selfie effect. JAMAFacialPlastSurg 2018;20:333–5.
10. Punthakee X, Rival R, Solomon P. Digital imaging in rhinoplasty. AestheticPlastSurg 2009;33:635–8.
11. Lohuis PJFM. Rhinoplasty analysis. In: Lohuis PJFM, editor. Advanced caucasian and mediterraneanrhinoplasty. Gilsum (NH): Kugler Publications; 2014. p. 43–68.
12. Byrd HS, Hobar PC. Rhinoplasty: a practical guide for surgical planning. PlastReconstr Surg 1993;91:642–54 [discussion: 655–6].
13. Rohrich RJ, Huynh B, Muzaffar AR, et al. Importance of the depressor septinasi muscle in rhinoplasty: anatomic study and clinical application. PlastReconstrSurg 2000;105:376–83.
14. Cachay-Velasquez H, Laguinge RE. Aesthetic treatment of the columella. Ann PlastSurg 1989;22:370–9.
15. Ebrahimi A, Nejadsarvari N, Motamedi MH, et al. Anatomic variations found on dissection of depressor septinasi muscles in cadavers. Arch FacialPlastSurg 2012;14:31–3.
16. Ho Y, Deeb R, Westreich R, et al. Effect of depressor septi resection in rhinoplasty on upper lip length. JAMAFacialPlastSurg 2014;16:272–6.
17. Kridel RW, Castellano RD. A simplified approach to alar base reduction: a review of 124 patients over 20 years. Arch FacialPlastSurg 2005;7:81–93.
18. Daniel RK. Middle Eastern rhinoplasty in the United States: Part I. Primary rhinoplasty. PlastReconstrSurg 2009;124:1630–9.
19. Berghaus A. Modern rhinoplasty: is there a place for the closed approach? FacialPlastSurg 2016;32:402–8.
20. Daniel RK. Middle Eastern rhinoplasty in the United States: Part II. Secondary rhinoplasty. PlastReconstrSurg 2009;124:1640–8.
21. Pereira Nunes D, Tinoco C, Oliveira ECD, et al. Intermediate osteotomies in rhinoplasty: a new perspective. Eur Arch Otorhinolaryngol 2017;274:2953–8.

22. Wright WK. Principles of nasal septum reconstruction. Trans Am AcadOphthalmolOtolaryngol 1969;73:252–5.
23. Lawson W, Westreich R. Correction of caudal deflections of the nasal septum with a modified Goldman septoplasty technique: how we do it. EarNoseThroat J 2007; 86:617–20.
24. Saharia PS, Deepti S. Septoplasty can change the shape of the nose. Indian J OtolaryngolHeadNeckSurg 2013;65:220–5.
25. Most SP. Anterior septal reconstruction: outcomes after a modified extracorporeal septoplasty technique. Arch FacialPlastSurg 2006;8:202–7.
26. King ED, Ashley FL. The correction of the internally and externally deviated nose. PlastReconstrSurg(1946) 1952;10:116–20.
27. Samaha M, Rassouli A. Spreader graft placement in endonasalrhinoplasty: Technique and a review of 100 cases. PlastSurg(Oakv) 2015;23:252–4.
28. Gunter JP, Friedman RM. Lateral crural strut graft: technique and clinical applications in rhinoplasty. PlastReconstrSurg 1997;99:943–52.
29. Rohrich RJ, Raniere J Jr, Ha RY. The alar contour graft: correction and prevention of alar rim deformities in rhinoplasty. PlastReconstrSurg 2002;109: 2495–505.
30. Rohrich RJ, Kurkjian TJ, Hoxworth RE, et al. The effect of the columellar strut graft on nasal tip position in primary rhinoplasty. PlastReconstrSurg 2012;130: 926–32.
31. Foda HM, Kridel RW. Lateral crural steal and lateral crural overlay: an objective evaluation. Arch OtolaryngolHeadNeckSurg 1999;125:1365–70.
32. Patrocinio LG, Patrocinio TG, Barreto DM, et al. Evaluation of lateral crural steal in nasal tip surgery. JAMAFacialPlastSurg 2014;16:400–4.
33. Alharethy S. Preferred nasolabial angle in Middle Eastern population. Eur Arch Otorhinolaryngol 2017;274:2339–41.
34. Pastorek NJ, Bustillo A, Murphy MR, et al. The extended columellar strut-tip graft. Arch FacialPlastSurg 2005;7:176–84.
35. Erol OO. Tip rhinoplasty in broad noses in a Turkish population: Eurasian noses. PlastReconstrSurg 2012;130:185–97.
36. Toriumi DM. New concepts in nasal tip contouring. Arch FacialPlastSurg 2006;8: 156–85.
37. Toriumi DM, Checcone MA. New concepts in nasal tip contouring. FacialPlastSurgClin North Am 2009;17:55–90, vi.
38. Gruber RP, Grover S. The anatomic tip graft for nasal augmentation. PlastReconstrSurg 1999;103:1744–53.
39. Quatela VC, Jacono AA. Structural grafting in rhinoplasty. FacialPlastSurg 2002; 18:223–32.
40. Gunter JP, Landecker A, Cochran CS. Frequently used grafts in rhinoplasty: nomenclature and analysis. PlastReconstrSurg 2006;118:14e–29e.
41. Powell N, Humphries B. Proportions of the aesthetic face. New York: Thieme-Stratton Inc; 1984.
42. Azizzadeh B, Mashkevich G. Middle Eastern rhinoplasty. FacialPlastSurgClin North Am 2010;18:201–6.
43. Benlier E, Top H, Aygit AC. A new approach to smiling deformity: cutting of the superior part of the orbicularis oris. AestheticPlastSurg 2005;29:373–7.
44. Lawson W, Reino AJ. Reduction columelloplasty.A new method in the management of the nasal base. Arch OtolaryngolHeadNeckSurg 1995;121:1086–8.
45. Fred GB. Role of depressor septinasi muscle in rhinoplasty. AMA Arch Otolaryngol 1955;62:37–41.

46. Hwang K, Kim DJ, Hwang G. Relationship between depressor septinasi muscle and dermocartilagenous ligament; anatomic study and clinical application. J CraniofacSurg 2006;17:286–90.
47. Surowitz JB, Most SP. Complications of rhinoplasty. FacialPlastSurgClin North Am 2013;21:639–51.
48. Holt GR, Garner ET, McLarey D. Postoperative sequelae and complications of rhinoplasty. OtolaryngolClin North Am 1987;20:853–76.
49. Hafezi F, Naghibzadeh B, Nouhi A. Management of the thick-skinned nose: a more effective approach. Ann OtolRhinolLaryngol 2006;115:444–9.
50. Ozucer B, Yildirim YS, Veyseller B, et al. Effect of postrhinoplasty taping on postoperative edema and nasal draping: a randomized clinical trial. JAMAFacialPlastSurg 2016;18:157–63.
51. Bhangoo KS. Aesthetic rhinoplasty: avoiding unfavourable results. Indian J PlastSurg 2013;46:349–58.
52. Wright WK. Symposium: the supra-tip in rhinoplasty: a dilemma. II. Influence of surrounding structure and prevention. Laryngoscope 1976;86:50–2.
53. Hanasono MM, Kridel RW, Pastorek NJ, et al. Correction of the soft tissue pollybeak using triamcinolone injection. Arch FacialPlastSurg 2002;4:26–30.

The Changing Face of America

Kate O'Connor, MD[a,b], Anthony E. Brissett, MD[b,*]

KEYWORDS

- Rhinoplasty • Ethnicity • Race • African American • Asian • Hispanic

KEY POINTS

- The proportion of nonwhite patients seeking rhinoplasty is increasing. As this population increases, the rhinoplasty surgeon has to be well adapted to diverse goals.
- Surgery has evolved from cultural transformation, in which the characteristics unique to a patient's ethnicity were altered to achieve a classically Western nose; to cultural restoration, when revision surgeries were performed to restore those qualities; and to finally arriving at cultural preservation and the union of unique features and facial harmony.
- Patients' self-identified ethnicity should be elicited in the consultation because ethnicity, race, and identity can be more complex than at first glance. Knowledge of a patient's self-image helps guide the consultation and align the patient's goals with the surgical outcome.

INTRODUCTION: THE US POPULATION TODAY

Since the birth of the nation, the US population has grown year after year. Based on the most recent 2018 estimations, the US population has grown to more than 329 million people, which represents a 6% increase from the 2010 census.[1] The official census takes place in 2020, but predictions are consistent with further growth. Looking beyond the next census and into the decades to follow, the US population is expected to exceed 439 million people in 2050.[2,3] As the population grows, racial and ethnic demographics also will continue to change.

Over the years, data acquisition and reporting for the US census have evolved in order to keep pace with changing demographics; 1960 marked the first time citizens could select their own racial identity.[4] The options for selection have increased from 2 races in the initial 1790 census to 6 racial categories, with 15 options in the most recent census.[4] Importantly, for the first time, in the 2000 census, individuals could

[a] Baylor College of Medicine, Department of Otolaryngology, 1977 Butler Blvd Suite E5.200 5th floor, Houston, TX 77030, USA; [b] Department Otolaryngology/Head and Neck Surgery, Division of Facial Plastic and Reconstructive Surgery, Texas A&M University College of Medicine, Houston Methodist ENT Specialists, 6550 Fannin Street, Suite 1703, Houston, TX 77030, USA
* Corresponding author.
E-mail address: aebrissett@houstonmethodist.org

Otolaryngol Clin N Am 53 (2020) 299–308
https://doi.org/10.1016/j.otc.2019.12.009
0030-6665/20/© 2020 Elsevier Inc. All rights reserved.

select more than 1 race, and 2.9% of the population elected to choose more than 1 race.[4]

Based on 2018 data, 60.7% of the population self-identified as white compared with 72% of individuals in the 2010 census.[5] The percentage of US citizens who identify as white is expected to decrease in decades to come and may fall below 50% by 2050, for the first time in US history.[2] Currently, the second-largest racial group is composed of people of Latino or Hispanic descent; 18.1% of the population reported being of Hispanic/Latino descent in the most recent 2018 estimate.[1] This was an approximate 2% increase from the 2010 census, when 16.3% identified as Hispanic or Latino[5]; 2050 predictions indicate that approximately 30% of the US population will be Hispanic or Latino, the largest growth rate among all racial groups.[2,3] Based on the same census estimates, 13.1% identified as black or African American in 2018 compared with 12.6% of the population in 2010.[1,5] The percentage of persons identifying as black or African American is expected to increase to 14% by 2050.[2] The percentage of the population identified as Asian was 5.8% in 2018 compared with 5.6% in 2010.[1,5] In 2050, people of Asian descent are predicted to account for approximately 9% of the US population.[2] Additionally, the 2010 census allowed for a write-in section, with 7% of the population selecting "some other race."[5] The opportunity to identify with more than 1 ethnicity in official government metrics is critical as the multiracial landscape of US citizens continues to evolve.

Additionally, as immigration rates have increased, so have multiracial marriages; 17% of newlyweds in the United States report being married to someone of a different race, representing a more than 500% increase compared with rates of mulitracial marriage in 1980.[6] With this in mind, the number of multiracial newborns subsequently has increased 3-fold since 1980.[6] In 2015, approximately 14% of US infants were multiracial.[7] Against this background, ethnic and racial awareness of patients is essential for the facial plastic surgeons employing the concepts of racial preservation in rhinoplasty surgery.

AESTHETIC SURGERY: MORE PREVALENT THAN EVER

Based on estimates from the American Society of Plastic Surgeons (ASPS), 17.5 million cosmetic procedures and 1.8 million cosmetic surgeries were performed in 2018.[8] The number of cosmetic procedures continues to rise, bolstered by the expanded popularity of neuromodulators, injectables, and other minimally invasive office-based procedures.[8] Botox (Allergan; Dublin, Ireland) injections have increased 22% since 2013. The number of cosmetic surgeries has doubled during that same time.[9] In 2018, the most popular surgeries included breast augmentation, liposuction, rhinoplasty, and blepharoplasty.[8] Rhinoplasty was the most commonly performed facial plastic surgery followed by blepharoplasty and rhytidectomy.[8,9] Based on the available ASPS data, at least 213,780 rhinoplasties were performed in 2018. Approximately three-fourths of rhinoplasty patients are female, but rhinoplasty is the most commonly performed facial plastic surgery for male patients.[10] Variances in cosmetic procedures exist across races, but rhinoplasty is the only surgery that is in the top 3 most commonly performed surgeries in white, Latino, African American, and Asian patients.[10–12] Rhinoplasty remains one of the top surgeries across all ethnicities for the last 15 years.

As demonstrated by census data, the population is diversifying, and the trend continues among patients seeking cosmetic surgery. In 2007, nonwhite patients accounted for 22% of all cosmetic procedures.[13] Currently, 30% of cosmetic procedures are performed on nonwhite patients.[11] When evaluating the number of cosmetic procedures based on ethnicity, patients of Hispanic or Latino descent represent the most common group behind whites. In 2017, Hispanic patients underwent 1.9 million cosmetic procedures, accounting for almost 11% of all cosmetic procedures performed. This total reflects a 16% increase from 2016.[11] The increase in Hispanic patients seeking cosmetic procedures has been a decades-long trend, as there was a 323% increase at the turn of the twenty-first century.[14]

In 2017, patients who identify as black or African American underwent approximately 1.6 million cosmetic procedures, representing 9% of all procedures performed. The number of procedures performed on black/African American patients shows a 17% percent increase from the year prior.[11] From 1999 to 2001, there was a reported 340% increase in African American patients requesting cosmetic procedures[14]; 6% of reported rhinoplasties performed in 2017 were performed on patients of African descent.[8,11] In 2017, Asian American patients underwent 1.2 million cosmetic procedures, which was unchanged from the previous year, accounting for 7% of all cosmetic procedures and 4% of rhinoplasties.[11] All other unspecified races, including those of Middle Eastern descent, were evaluated together and represented approximately 500,000 cosmetic procedures, in 2017. Compared with 2016, there was a 38% percent decrease in the number of procedures performed on this subgroup.[11] The decrease could be representative for a change in patient demand, or patients may have changing preferences regarding where their surgery is performed.

Based on current trends, cosmetic procedures likely will continue to increase in popularity across ages, genders, and races. Surgery is discussed more readily in conversation and is portrayed on television and on social media platforms. Given the increasing diversity of the United States, the diversity of patients should continue to increase as well. Understanding of different races, their cultures, and aesthetic ideals will be critical.

RACE, ETHNICITY, AND SELF-IDENTITY

The concepts of race, culture, and ethnicity are challenging to define and frequently have changed over time, depending on context. For many centuries, *race* referred to a group of people with a common ancestor or homeland and was used similarly to the use of the word, *nationality*, today.[15–17] In the 1700s, the definition shifted from ancestral to physical commonalities. Race then represented a predetermined, biological distinction between individuals and groups. For centuries to follow, race often was the justification for both phenotypic and cultural differences and discrimination.[18] Today, race is built on its etymology and refers to a distinct population within the human species.[19] That population may be based on unique physical characteristics compared with another population, particularly when describing a group outside of the self. Race also may be used to identify a population with a separate, unifying culture or history.[19] The US Census Bureau defines race as a "person's self-identification with one or more social group."[20] This definition's use of "social group" intersects with concepts of culture, heritage, ethnicity, and self-identity. It is reflective of the evolving concepts regarding race and heritage, particularly in the setting of multiethnicity.

Definitions remain challenging because ethnicity and race often are used interchangeably despite subtle differences. *Ethnicity* typically refers to a population with a common history and cultural practices that differentiates the group from other populations.[21] Its definition functions similarly to how race was used in the 1500s. Today, ethnicity often replaces race as a more socially acceptable descriptor.[16,17] This shift highlights the important role social norms play in defining complex concepts, such as these.

Because these concepts rest so heavily on identity, experiences, social trends, and geopolitical events, the authors propose a distinction that is centered on the perception of the individual. It is the authors' hope that this distinction adds clarity to defining these terms within the context of patients. Race refers to how people/others view an individual; it can be a list of nationalities, physical attributes, and cultures a person inherits. Ethnicity is how individuals view themselves and the group they choose to identify with. This delineation regarding who is doing the defining has important implications for how individuals experience their reality, particularly if their ethnic identity deviates from what an outsider is expecting. This concept of ethnic self-identification becomes significant when considering self-image, concepts of beauty, and ethnic preservation during evaluation for facial plastic surgery, in particular rhinoplasty.

An example of this concept is a comparison and contrast between Tiger Woods and Barack Obama, two men of enormous talent and societal importance who both have reached the pinnacle of their respective careers. Beyond accolades and public recognition, there are cultural similarities between the two: both are of multiracial descent. Based on appearance, people describe both of these men as black or African American men, yet their identities and preferences are not congruent. Tiger Woods describes himself as cablinasian—a word he created in childhood to describe his white, black, Indian, and Asian heritage.[22] To Woods, his Asian heritage is extremely influential and takes into consideration the cultural and racial contributions of his maternal ancestry. It is essential in how he views himself and to define him singularly as black diminishes the importance he places on his multiracial heritage. Barack Obama, on the other hand, is of African and white descent, and, in contrast to Woods, he identifies uniformly with the African American diaspora.[23] Both Woods and Obama have had life experiences that have shaped how they define their multiethnicity and that certainly have had an impact on their sense of self, self-image, and concepts of attractiveness.

Woods, Obama, and millions of US citizens who have multiracial roots are shaped not only by their genome but also by family life, community, and life experiences that make up the culture around them. Although there are examples of overarching cultural trends, surgeons must pay attention to the patient present in the consultation room. A seemingly confident patient may struggle with self-esteem and feelings of falling short of perceived beauty ideals. Likewise, it is foolish to presume a patient is self-conscious about a particular facial feature. Self-confidence then arises from a strong sense of self and an absence of conflict with self-identity. These concepts depend on each other to create a healthy mental state (**Fig. 1**). Presumptions about a patient's self-confidence and aesthetic goals can be even more hazardous when the surgeon and patient are of differing racial identities as the lenses may differ.

Patients presenting for consultation undoubtedly have their own preferences and identities, shaped by the themes discussed previously. It is important for facial plastic surgeons to recognize that patients may have ethnic identities that do not appear to align with their projected race. Asking patients which ethnicity they identify with is the most authentic, direct, and facile way to ensure the consultation fosters rapport and that surgical outcomes align with a patient's desired results.

TRANSFORMATION TO PRESERVATION

For many years, the goals of rhinoplasty surgery were to change the nose in an attempt to mirror the classic neocanon and Western leptorrhine ideals with little nuance or consideration of race or culture. Surgical outcomes often resulted in a complete cultural transformation. After transformative rhinoplasty, physical features often

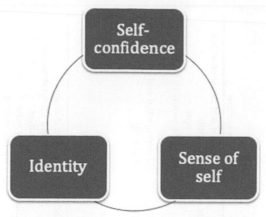

Fig. 1. Interplay and interdependence of personal identity, sense of self, and self-confidence.

no longer are congruent with how patients view themselves and how the world may view them. The postoperative outcome often is disharmonious with their other cultural or ethnic facial features.

Over time, the perspective of rhinoplasty surgeons and the expected outcomes of ethnically diverse patients have evolved. A shift from cultural transformation to cultural preservation has been witnessed, with the postsurgical goal of harmonizing and complementing and enhancing unique racial features rather than eliminating them.[24] Many investigators echo these sentiments.[13,14,25–27] When considering rhinoplasty in any patient, the current paradigm should include exploring a patient's personal thoughts and awareness of ethnicity and proceed with discussions that champion the preservation of ethnic characteristics. The authors encourage the process of moving away from definitions and associations of varying ethnicities and instead focusing on the anatomic characteristics involved in the nose of the patient present in clinic.[14,28–31]

To further emphasize that the concept of preservation spans all races, how frequently does a patient state, "after surgery, I still want to look like me" during a consultation? In general, rhinoplasty patients want to improve their appearance while at the same time preserving their unique features in a way that enhances facial harmony. Aesthetic concerns of the individual must be emphasized and addressed regardless of a patient's ethnic or racial ideal, and a clear discussion with patients about their goals is paramount. When consulting with patients who are of varying ethnicities, additional time to clarify preferences and goals must be taken into consideration.

NASAL ASSESSMENT

Investigators debate if universal truths of beauty and attractiveness are constant across cultures[32] or if a culture has its own standards.[33] Some investigators question the utility of using race and ethnicity in rhinoplasty at all.[16] The truth lies somewhere in the middle; symmetry, a trend toward averageness, and sexual dimorphism of facial features[34–38] result in a generally attractive face across all races and sexes. What is celebrated as beautiful, however, may vary among cultures.

Given its central position, a harmonious nose fades into the background whereas a distracting nose detracts from a face that otherwise may be composed of aesthetically

Table 1
Nasal assessment among nonwhite patients

	Hispanic	African American	Asian	Middle Eastern
Anatomic characteristics	Thick soft tissue envelope	Short nose	Short nose	Variable soft tissue envelope
	Low radix	Thick soft tissue envelope	Thick soft tissue envelope	High radix
	Short, weak nasal bones	Shorter, flatter nasal bones	Low radix	Longer nose
	Low, wide dorsum, possible hump	Low, widened dorsum—may be concave or saddled	Low dorsum	High dorsum with hump (often bony)
	Weak upper lateral cartilages	Broad middle vault with collapse	Wide alar base	Overprojected and over-rotated
	Wide alar base with weak ala	Wide alar base with strong ala	Weak lower lateral cartilage	Ptotic tip
	Wide lower lateral cartilage	Caudally oriented lower lateral cartilage	Horizontally oriented nostril	
	Bulbous tip	Bulbous, amorphous tip	Bulbous, rounded tip	
	Underprojected	Variable columellar length	Short columella	
	Short columella	Underprojected maxilla		
	Maxillary protrusion			
Average patient desires	Narrower dorsum	Straight, narrower dorsum	Increase dorsal height and projection	Straight dorsum
	Increased dorsal projection	Increased dorsal projection	Increased tip rotation, definition, and projection	Increased tip rotation and definition
	Increased tip definition and projection	Increased tip definition and projection		Shorter nose
	Narrowed base	Decreased alar flare		Tip refinement

pleasing features. Although the characteristics of the nose and underlying anatomy may vary, the overall desired outcomes are universal. Patients want a straight nose, appropriately sized and free of asymmetries, that does not distract from the rest of their face. When evaluating the unique nasal features of patients of ethnic descent, it is clear that there are no attributes that can be applied uniformly. In general, however, when discussing patients of ethnic descent seeking rhinoplasty procedures, there often are several features and desires that can be applied frequently.

Hispanic patients seeking rhinoplasty procedures have a tendency to have a thicker soft tissue envelope compared with their leptorrhine counterparts. The nasal bones often are shorter and the septal and alar cartilage may be less abundant with decreased inherent strength in Hispanic patients seeking nasal refinement.[39–41] The dorsum of Hispanic patients seeking nasal surgery can be either overprojected or underprojected. The alar base often is wider with less projection, and definition with the anterior nasal spine may be less prominent, resulting in a more acute nasolabial angle.[39–41] Hispanic patients seeking rhinoplasty procedures tend to desire refinement. Depending on appearance and demographics, there may be a need for either reduction or augmentation. Generally speaking, there often is a need to refine the nasal tip by increasing nasal tip projection, narrowing the alar base, and improving nasal tip definition.[39,40] A similar profile and desired outcome can be seen in patients of African and Asian descent seeking rhinoplasty procedures[27,42–47] **(Table 1)**. There may be variances in the strength and orientation of the lower lateral cartilages, the degree of maxillary projection, and columellar length.

For Middle Eastern patients seeking rhinoplasty, their soft tissue envelope can be either thick or thin. A dorsal contour irregularity involving both the bony and cartilaginous structures often is present rhinoplasty.[48–50] In this ethnic subgroup, the nasal tip often is overprojected, ptotic, and over-rotated. Patients from the Middle East seeking nasal surgery most often desire nasal reduction and refinement.[48–50]

When considering rhinoplasty in patients of varying ethnicities, contemporary thought has shifted away from ethnic or cultural transformation to one of preservation; a philosophy that supports maintaining the characteristics that are unifying to their ethnicity culture while enhancing their unique features and appearance is a superior approach.

SUMMARY

As the US population continues to grow and diversify, the cultural demographics continue to evolve in tandem. With this shift, it is recognized that the nonwhite population is increasing, and patients are more likely to be multiracial. The prominence and acceptance of aesthetic surgery are growing as well. Therefore, when evaluating patients for rhinoplasty, it is essential that the rhinoplasty surgeon be aware of the interplay of race, ethnicity, and self-image when considering patients' desires and expected outcomes. Coupling the knowledge of a patient's ethnic identity with the patient's desires allows for preservation surgery that highlights features in a harmonious way. Rhinoplasty has never been a 1-size-fits-all surgery, and, with the changing face of America, it will continue to be an individualized arrangement between patient and surgeon.

REFERENCES

1. United States Census Bureau. Quick facts United States. Available at: https://www.census.gov/quickfacts/fact/table/US/PST045218. Accessed June 21, 2019.

2. Passel J, Cohn D. U.S. population projections: 2005-2050. Pew Research Center; 2008. Available at: https://www.pewsocialtrends.org/2008/02/11/us-population-projections-2005-2050/. Accessed June 7, 2019.

3. Cohn D. Future immigration will change the face of America by 2065. Pew Research Center; 2015. Available at: https://www.pewresearch.org/fact-tank/2015/10/05/future-immigration-will-change-the-face-of-america-by-2065/. Accessed July 1, 2019.

4. Pew Research Center. What census calls us: a historical timeline 2015. Available at: https://www.pewsocialtrends.org/interactives/multiracial-timeline/. Accessed July 1, 2019.

5. United States Census Bureau. 2010 Census shows America's diversity. 2011. Available at: https://www.census.gov/newsroom/releases/archives/2010_census/cb11-cn125.html. Accessed June 1, 2019.

6. Livingtsong G, Brown A. Interracial marriage in the U.S 50 years after Loving v Virginia. Pew Research Center; 2017. Available at: https://www.pewsocialtrends.org/2017/05/18/intermarriage-in-the-u-s-50-years-after-loving-v-virginia/. Accessed July 5, 2019.

7. Livingston G. The rise of multiracial and multiethnic babies in the U.S. Pew Research Center. Available at: https://www.pewresearch.org/fact-tank/2017/06/06/the-rise-of-multiracial-and-multiethnic-babies-in-the-u-s/June 6 2017. Accessed July 6, 2019.

8. American Society of Plastic Surgeons. Plastic surgery statistics 2018. Available at: https://www.plasticsurgery.org/documents/News/Statistics/2018/plastic-surgery-statistics-report-2018.pdf.

9. International Communications Research. AAFPRS Membership Study. Conducted for the American Academy of facial plastic and Reconstructive surgery. International Communication Survey; 2018. Available at: http://www.icrsurvey.com. Accessed June 20, 2019.

10. International Communications Research. AAFPRS Membership Study. Conducted for the American Academy of Facial Plastic and Reconstructive Surgery. International Communication Survey; 2011. Available at: http://www.icrsurvey.com. Accessed June 20, 2019.

11. American Society of Plastic Surgeons. 2017 Plastic surgery statistics report 2018. Available at: https://www.plasticsurgery.org/documents/News/Statistics/2017/cosmetic-procedures-ethnicity-2017.pdf. Accessed June 1, 2019.

12. Cobo R. Structural rhinoplasty in Latin American patients. Facial Plast Surg 2013;29:171–83.

13. Wimalawansa S, McKnight A, Bullocks JM. Socioeconomic impact of ethnic cosmetic surgery: trends and potential financial impact the African American, Asian American, Latin American, and Middle Eastern communities have on cosmetic surgery. Semin Plast Surg 2009;23(3):159–62.

14. Sturm-O'Brien AK, Brissett AE. Ethnic trends in facial plastic surgery. Facial Plast Surg 2010;26(2):69–74.

15. Stamper K. Why we confuse race and ethnicity: a lexicographer's perspective. Conscious Style Guide. Available at: https://consciousstyleguide.com/why-we-confuse-race-ethnicity-lexicographers-perspective/. Feb 13 2019. Accessed July 17, 2019.

16. Leong SC, Eccles R. Race and ethnicity in nasal plastic surgery: a need for science. Facial Plast Surg 2010;26(02):063–8.

17. Spencer S. Race and ethnicity: culture, identity and representation. New York: Routledge; 2006. Available at: http://armytage.net/pdsdata/[Stephen_Spencer]_Race_and_Ethnicity_Identity,_Cu(BookFi.org).pdf.

18. Goodman A. Reflections on "race" in science and society in the United States. J Anthropol Sci 2017;95:283–90.

19. "Race." Merriam-Webster.com. 2011. Available at: https://www.merriam-webster.com/dictionary/race. Accessed June 2, 2019.

20. United States Census Bureau. Race and ethnicity. United States Department of Commerce. Economics, and Statistics Application; 2017. Available at: https://www.census.gov/mso/www/training/pdf/race-ethnicity-onepager.pdf. Accessed July 9 2019.

21. Barth F. Enduring and emerging issues in the analysis of ethnicity. The anthropology of ethnicity, H Vermulen, CGovers. Amsterdam: Het Spinhuis; 1996.

22. Wise M. Serena Williams, Tiger Woods, and racial identity in sports. ESPN. Available at: https://www.espn.com/tennis/story/_/id/13551475/tiger-woods-serena-williams-racial-identity. Aug 31, 2015. Accessed August 1, 2019.

23. Coates Ta-Nehisi. 'It's what we do more than what we say:' Obama on race, identity and the way forward. The Atlantic. Available at: https://www.theatlantic.com/politics/archive/2016/12/ta-nehisi-coates-obama-transcript-iii/511475/. December 22 2016. Accessed on July 24, 2019.

24. Flowers RS. The surgical correction of the non-Caucasian nose. Clin Plast Surg 1977;4(1):69–87.

25. Wang TD. Non-Caucasian rhinoplasty. Facial Plast Surg 2003;19(3):247–56.

26. Kridel RW, Rowe-Jones J. Ethnicity in facial plastic surgery. Facial Plast Surg 2010;26(2):61–2.

27. Lam S, Revision rhinoplasty for the Asian nose. Facial Plast Surg; 24(3):372-377

28. Thomas JR, Dixon TK. A global perspective of beauty in a multicultural world. JAMA Facial Plast Surg 2016;18(1):7–8.

29. Stucker FJ. Non-Caucasian rhinoplasty and adjunctive reduction cheiloplasty. Otolaryngol Clin North Am 1987;20:877–94.

30. Rohrich RJ, Bolden K. Ethnic rhinoplasty. Clin Plast Surg 2010;37:353–70.

31. Kridel RWH. Commentary on lower lateral cartilages: an anatomic and morphological study in the noses of black southern Africans." Aesthet Surg J 2017; 37(3):283–4.

32. Sands NB, Adamson PA. Global facial beauty: approaching a unified aesthetic ideal. Facial Plast Surg 2014;30(2):93–100.

33. Bashour M. History and current concepts in the analysis of facial attractiveness. Plast Reconstr Surg 2006;118(3):741–56.

34. Rhodes G. The evolutionary psychology of facial beauty. Annu Rev Psychol 2006; 57(1):199–226.

35. Weeks DM, Thomas JR. Beauty in a multicultral world. Facial Plast Surg Clin North Am 2014;22(3):337–41.

36. Grinfeld A, Betelli R, Arruda G, et al. How to harmonize the ethnic Nose. Facial Plast Surg 2016;32(6):620–4.

37. Tai C. Fall 2019 runway diversity report: racial and age diversity step forward, size and gender inclusivity a step back. The Fashion spot. Available at: https://www.thefashionspot.com/runway-news/828413-diversity-report-fall-2019-runways/ October 25 2019. Accessed July 2, 2019.

38. Matory WE, Falces E. Non-Caucasian rhinoplasty : a 16-year experience. Plast Reconstr Surg 1986;77(2):239–51.

39. Cobo R. Rhinoplasty in latino patients. Clin Plast Surg 2016;43(1):237–54.

40. Milgrim LM, Lawson W, Cohen AF. Anthropometric Analysis of Female Latino noses: Revised aesthetic concepts and their surgical implications. Arch Otolaryngol Head Neck Surg 1996;122(10):1079–86.
41. Cobo R. Facial aesthetic surgery with emphasis on rhinoplasty in the Hispanic patient. Curr Opin Otolaryngol Head Neck Surg 2008;16(4):369–74.
42. Ofodile FA, Bokhari F, Ellis C. The black American nose. Ann Plast Surg 1993; 31(3):209–18.
43. Rohrick RJ, Muzaffar AR. Rhinoplasty in the African-American Patient. Plast Reconstr Surg 2003;111(3):1322–39.
44. Rees TD. Nasal plastic surgery in the negro. Plast Reconstr Surg 1969; 43(1):13–8.
45. Snyder G. Rhinoplasty in the negro. Annual Meeting of American Society of Plastic Surgeons. Atlanta, GA, Feb 2, 1970.
46. Toriumi DM, Swartout B. Asian rhinoplasty. Facial Plast Surg Clin North Am 2007; 15(3):293–307.
47. Boyette JR, Stucker FJ. African American rhinoplasty. Facial Plast Surg Clin North Am 2014;22:279–393.
48. Rohrich RJ, Ghavami A. Rhinoplasty for Middle Eastern noses. Plast Reconstr Surg 2009;123:1343–54.
49. Daniel RK. Middle Eastern rhinoplasty: anatomy, aesthetics, and surgical planning. Facial Plast Surg 2010;26:110–8.
50. Pourdanesh F, Tabrizi R, Vahedi R, et al. Ethnic rhinoplasty in Iranians: the oral and maxillofacial surgery experience. J Oral Maxillofac Surg 2014;72: 2568.e1-7.

Management of the Nasal Tip, Nasal Base, and Soft Tissue Envelope in Patients of African Descent

Kofi D.O. Boahene, MD

KEYWORDS

• Ethnic sensitive rhinoplasty • African American rhinoplasty • African rhinoplasty

KEY POINTS

• Among patients of African descent, there is a strong desire for maintaining nasal features that are ethnically sensitive and culturally congruent.
• The core rhinoplasty techniques, framework exposure, cartilage grafting, suture contouring and repositioning, and osteotomies are universal when performing rhinoplasty regardless of ethnicity.
• The nasal skin envelope in the African patient is a key determinant in rhinoplasty outcomes. The thick nasal skin can be delicately and precisely debulked to soften its stiffness and allow better coaptation and improved contouring.
• Highly projected nasal tips are ethnically incongruent among Africans; tip projection should be performed in a measured manner.

INTRODUCTION

The facial structure, nasal shape, and aesthetic nasal preferences vary broadly among patients of African descent who seek rhinoplasty. This variation is a reflection of the broad diversity in this ethnic group and is highlighted by the lapses in computer vision algorithms in accurately recognizing black faces. All the same, across ethnicities, patients who seek rhinoplasty have similar goals: a reshaped nose that fits their facial features and enhances their facial beauty. Among patients of African descent, there is a particularly strong desire for maintaining nasal features that are ethnically sensitive and culturally congruent. Surgeons must be well vexed with these sensitivities when approaching rhinoplasty in this group. A working concept of what is deemed ethnically sensitive and culturally congruent is gained from analyzing noses of Africans who have

Otolaryngology Head and Neck Surgery, Division of Facial Plastic and Reconstructive Surgery, Department of Otolaryngology Head and Neck Surgery, The Johns Hopkins University School of Medicine, Johns Hopkins Outpatient Center, 601 N. Caroline St, 6th Floor, Baltimore, MD 21287, USA
E-mail address: dboahen1@jhmi.edu

Otolaryngol Clin N Am 53 (2020) 309–317
https://doi.org/10.1016/j.otc.2019.12.007

oto.theclinics.com

had no previous rhinoplasties and feedback from patients seeking primary or revision rhinoplasty. The core rhinoplasty techniques, framework exposure, cartilage grafting, suture contouring and repositioning, and osteotomies are universal when performing rhinoplasty regardless of ethnicity. Thus, it is the ethnically sensitive preferences and response of the African nose to these standard rhinoplasty maneuvers that introduces unique nuances when reshaping the African nose.[1]

The nasal tip is a central facial aesthetic feature and its modification a common reason Africans seek rhinoplasty. A beautiful nasal tip blends into the face despite its projected and central position. Studies of human gaze patterns using eye-tracking and visual scan paths have shown that observers track the human face in a stereotypical pattern of saccades and fixation that only transiently focuses on the nasal tip but longer on the eyes.[2,3] The nose should not become a core facial feature that visually stands out after rhinoplasty. An altered nasal tip, when harsh and unnatural in appearance, alters the normal visual scan path and attracts unwanted attention or comments ("they had a nose job"). Beyond appearance, the nasal tip is soft to touch and naturally mobile. The mobility and softness of the nasal tip is often sacrificed for a defined yet stiff tip, a source of discontent among some rhinoplasty patients.

Alar contour, nostril size, tip definition, and alar base width are the core aspects of the nasal tip addressed in African rhinoplasty.

ALAR CONTOURING AND NOSTRIL RESHAPING

On frontal view, the alar margin transitions from the nasal tip to the ala-facial groove as a smooth curvy line that visually and in photographs softly reflects light (**Fig. 1**). The alar margin is devoid of cartilage and its shape and contour is maintained by thick fibrous subcutaneous tissue. A slight dip at the level of the soft tissue triangle or a shadow line from the alar grove distinguishes the tip subunit from the ala subunit. A straight alar margin inserting on the cheek without much curvature, as described in distinctive white noses, is not typical in African noses. Rather, the alar characteristically curves to insert on the cheeks. A pronounced curvature, also described as alar

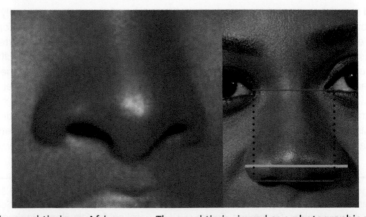

Fig. 1. The nasal tip in an African nose. The nasal tip is viewed as a photographic and visual reflection of highlights and shadows. The alar margin transitions from the tip-defining points as a smooth curvy line with a natural curve when inserting onto the cheek. The alar flare (*red lines*) is distinct from the alar base width (*green line*). In African nose, we find the intercaruncular distance a more natural measure of an appropriate alar base width than the intercanthal distance.

flare, when undesirable, is modified with various techniques. Additionally, alar flare, although a static feature, may be dynamically exaggerated when smiling. Patients often describe this as "my nose spreads when I smile." Patients with dynamic alar flare often avoid smiling in photographs. Curtailing the degree of dynamic flare minimizes nasal distortion in photographs when patients smile. The size, shape, and orientation of the nostrils are important when analyzing the nasal tip for aesthetic modification. The nostrils are bounded by the alar margins laterally, the soft tissue triangles superiorly, the columella medially, and the nasal sill inferiorly. Each of these anatomic boundaries are defined by underlying cartilage fibrous soft tissue. Alterations in any one of these substructures changes the shape, orientation, or size of the nostrils.

Static and Dynamic Alar Flare Reduction

The degree of alar flare is reduced with alar margin rim grafts, by projecting the nasal tip or by directly excising alar soft tissue. Alar rim grafts are placed directly along the alar margin for support against collapse or to correct alar margin asymmetries, mild notching, and retraction. A strong alar rim graft spanning a flared alar margin is able to modify the degree of curvature in a manner similar to the effect of a shirt collar stiffener.[4] Mild to moderate alar flare may be satisfactorily modified in this manner obviating alar base excisions (**Fig. 2**).

In patients with underprojected nasal tips, alar flare is reduced by projecting the central structural pillar of the tip tripod. This is technically achieved by various means all of which essentially lengthen the medial and intermediate crura. Overprojected nasal tips are, however, ethnically incongruent among Africans and should be applied In a measured manner.

Tip projection may be achieved by recruiting lateral crura or raising and fixating the medial and intermediate crura at a higher position on to a stable columella strut or a straight and stable nasal septum either directly or by an extended caudal septal graft. A stable central tip support minimizes secondary dynamic flaring when patients smile.

Lateral crura recruitment for tip projection is performed in various ways. One way is to completely release the lateral crus from the underlying vestibule, marking and creating a new laterally positioned dome with suture plication and then transposing

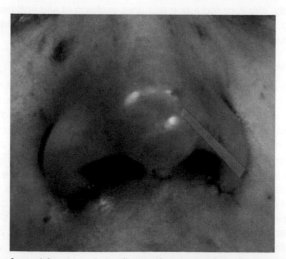

Fig. 2. Alar rim graft modification of alar flare. Alar rim grafting for correction of alar flare. (*Left*) Before alar rim grafting. (*Right*) After alar rim grafting.

the new dome medially to project the nasal tip.[5,6] This technique essentially shortens the effective length of the lateral crus, which if not compensated for can result in alar retraction or collapse. The shortened lateral crus is compensated for by placing a lateral crural strut that extends beyond the end of the shortened crus. Totally freeing the lateral crus from the underlying vestibule is not always necessary but allows the freed cartilage to be mobilized and transposed in an unrestricted and versatile manner. The lateral crura is transposed with the attached lining if their composite mobility is unrestricted.

Fixating the medial and intermediate crural cartilages on to a central cartilaginous pillar is an effective means of projecting the nasal tip and secondarily reducing nasal alar flare. Technically, the media and intermediate crural cartilages are separated and fixated higher on to a straight and strong columella strut placed between the them. If the medial crural footplates are overly long, they may be recruited centrally but should not be completely plicated because that distorts and widens the nostrils. The columella strut should be position just above the nasal spine leaving a structure-free zone of compression. As with the use of columella strut, the tip cartilages may be suspended on to the caudal edge of the nasal septum in a more projected position. This technique is effective in achieving a stable nasal tip but has attendant complexities that should be appreciated and accounted for. The caudal end of the nasal septum should be straight, in the midline long enough to allow transposition and fixation of the intermediate and medial crural cartilages without inappropriately shortening the nose or causing columella retraction. Long septal cartilages are, however, not typical in African noses. Thus, extending the effective length of the cartilaginous nasal septum with an extension graft is often necessary.[7,8] The caudal septal extension graft should be straight and stable because immediate or delayed displacement of the graft takes the tip with it. One major drawback in fixating the nasal tip on a caudal septum is the elimination of the natural compressibility of the membranous septum. The nasal tip is the most projected feature of the face and its softness and compressibility when touched is important. Eliminating this feeling of softness for specific aesthetic gains should be considered carefully. One way to maintain a sense of softness to the nasal tip is to preserve aspects of the membranous septum to allow compression when placing caudal septal extension grafts.

More commonly, alar flare reduction requires excision of alar soft tissue. Besides its effect on alar flap, alar soft tissue excision can affect the shape, orientation, and size of the nostrils (discussed next).

Alar Base Reduction and Nostril Reshaping

Wide alar base is a common reason patients of African descent seek rhinoplasty. The alar base width is distinct from alar flare and is measured as the distance between the two alar-facial transition points. The appropriate alar base width is determined from patient to patient based on the aesthetic proportions of the entire face. The alar base width is commonly analyzed in the context of midfacial width and intercanthal distance. The alar base is considered wide when the alar is positioned lateral to the medial canthi in whites. In patients of African descent, we find the intercaruncular width a better reference point than the intercanthal width. Alar base width reduction requires removal of tissue from the sill and repositioning of the alar base (**Fig. 3**).

To improve precision, the desired extent of alar base reduction should be determined and marked before any distortion from injections and swelling. We first measure the intercaruncular distance as a guide for how wide the alar base width should be. The difference between the intercaruncular distance and the alar base width is a rough guide to how much base reduction is needed. The major component of base reduction

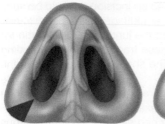
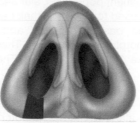
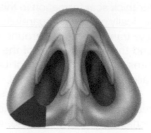

Fig. 3. Alar base reduction.

is achieved not from sill excision but from medial alar advancement into deeper tissue void created between the ala attachment and the nasal spine. The amount of sill excision is more relevant for nostril reduction and reshaping rather than base width reduction. Deep tissue excision and medial alar base advancement is done via a sublabial approach without any sill incision in cases when nostril size reduction is not necessary (see **Fig. 3**).

On base view, the nostril takes on a pearlike shape and can vary widely in size and orientation (**Fig. 1**). The nostrils are more commonly horizontally or obliquely oriented. A natural and ethnically congruent nostril shape is an extremely important aesthetic feature among African rhinoplasty patients. Maintaining the natural alar curvature and ovoid nostril shape is important to many patients seeking African American rhinoplasty. When nostril reduction and alar reshaping is planned, the final outcome should respect these natural curves and shapes. Poorly executed nostril reshaping is a common reason for patient dissatisfaction after African American rhinoplasty and should therefore be performed with careful planning and caution. The potential for nostril asymmetry despite meticulous effort should be discussed with patients before surgery.

When analyzing the alar and nostrils for reshaping, a problem-oriented approach is helpful. Is the alar base width wide? Is the alar flare pronounced? Are the nostrils wide? Are the nostrils asymmetric? What is the natural orientation of the nostrils? Answers to these questions can guide one in planning and selecting the appropriate technique when planning for alar base reduction and nostril reshaping in the African patient. Alar excisions are designed with incisions placed along the inner or outer aspects of the rim or as a full-thickness excision through the alar. Given the propensity

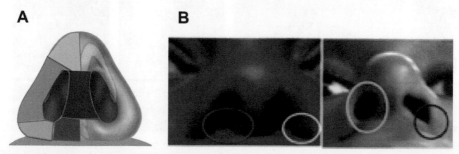

Fig. 4. Nostril reshaping. (*A*) Nasal base is conceptualized as having imaginary subunits (*color segments*) with transition points that are helpful when planning nostril reshaping techniques. (*B*) Poor nostril reduction outcomes (*red*). Effaced sill ridge (*yellow*). No alar curvature (*green*). Normal and (*blue*) notched sill.

for thick scar formation in this patient population, alar and sill incisions should be strategically placed and carefully closed to maximize their camouflage. There are discernible transition points around the "base-sill junction" and the junction between the sill and the lateral border of the footplates (see **Fig. 4**). These transition points are ideal sites to place incisions for base or nostril reduction. The shape of the excised sill is tailored to the desired goal.

Alar and nostril asymmetries and unnatural contours are among the most common reasons patients seek revision surgery. **Fig. 4**B shows examples of common distortions: the effaced sill ridge, no alar curvature, and notched sill. These complications are avoided with careful planning and a working understanding of what looks congruent on the African face. In planning and inspecting the nasal base before and after alar and nostril reshaping, it is helpful to visualize the alar nostril complex as having imaginary subunits (see **Fig. 4**). These subunits should match for symmetry to occur. Any preexisting nostril and alar asymmetry should be pointed out to the patient. Residual asymmetry is likely to persist even after careful attempt at correction.

TIP DEFINITION

Nasal tip definition is viewed as a visual phenomenon created by the contrast of light reflected off high points and shadow areas of light absorption.[8] Nasal tip–defining suturing and grafting techniques should be planned to establish light reflecting and absorbing contours. Nasal tip definition should not be considered synonymous with tip narrowness. The shape, strength, and contour of the tip cartilages and the thickness of the overlying skin particularly influence tip definition. If the tip is poorly defined, the contribution from the skin and tip cartilage contour is determined. Correcting bulbous tips resulting predominantly from thick skin is more challenging than that resulting from broad lower lateral cartilages and wide intradomal angles. The commonly used tip-defining suture and grafting techniques generally used in rhinoplasty are applicable in the African nose but their effect may be obscured when the skin is thick and but secondary scarring. Managing the thick skin and controlling the degree of scarring is discussed later.

Nasal tip surgery should be approached with the mindset of a structural engineer. The structural engineer considers the foundational needs of the construct and designs supporting pillars and beams that can withstand loading forces and external insults for a long time. Without adequate tip support, it is unlikely to achieve long-term tip

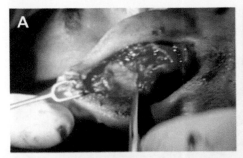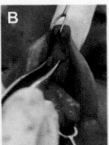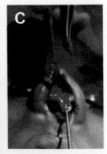

Fig. 5. The skin envelope is selectively debulked to achieve better contrast and definition from framework modification. The areas to be debulked should be precisely outlined before injection. Areas commonly debulked include the tip, supratip, and supra-alar regions. Selective debulking using (*A*) scissors and (*B*) forceps plucking technique. (*C*) Removed submuscular aponeurotic system.

definition in the African nose. Several of the tip-supporting techniques, such as the use of columella strut and caudal extension grafts, have previously been discussed. Although these structural grafts are effective, one should consider preserving as much as possible, and whenever feasible, the intrinsic tip supporting elements. This is achieved by carefully planning the surgical approach and limiting the extent of soft tissue dissection. It is helpful to be versatile in the use of endonasal and open structure rhinoplasty techniques.

SOFT TISSUE ENVELOPE

The secondary response and adaptation of the soft tissue envelope to technical modifications of the nasal tip cartilaginous framework determines the ultimate appearance and definition of the nasal tip. In African rhinoplasty, the soft tissue envelope is a dominant variable and a key determinant of rhinoplasty outcomes. African noses are typically described as thick skinned with abundant subcutaneous fibrofatty tissue. This generalized characterization fails to appreciate the broad variation in skin thickness among patients of African descent. When the nasal tip skin is moderately thick, the skin envelope responds to rhinoplasty in a predictable manner and does not require any special intervention. On the contrary, the severely thick nasal skin envelope obscures the contours of the underlying nasal substructure and reflects light uniformly as one unit without any contrasting shadows for tip definition. This skin type is likely oily, coarse in texture, and acne prone. It is common to express sebum from this skin type when tightly squeezed. The thick nasal skin contracts to adapt to framework changes slowly and is more likely to contribute to an amorphous nose if the framework is overly reduced.

Severely thick nasal skin envelope is challenging to refine but often requires specific modifications to achieve the nasal tip definition. Thick nasal skin contracts and adapts poorly to structural changes performed on the underlying framework. The propensity for postsurgical subcutaneous scarring effaces any potential definition gained from the typical tip-defining and grafting techniques. To overcome these challenges, surgeons often recommend large grafts or implants that put the skin on stretch to achieve definition. However, the definition achieved using these methods often results in a larger and more projected nose, which is often ethnically incongruent.

The thick nasal skin can be delicately and precisely debulked to soften its stiffness and allow better coaptation and improved contouring. Skin debulking should be performed selectively and not beyond the dermal plexus (see **Fig. 5**). With a scissor the subcutaneous fibrofatty tissue is bluntly dissected off while repeatedly palpating the skin to assess changes in pliability. The fibrofatty tissue can also be precisely debulked with plucking technique using an Adson-Brown forceps. The skin is aggressively debulked over the side walls cephalad to the alar crease by resecting the submuscular aponeurotic system (SMAS) layer. The immediate effect of debulking is evaluated visually and by pinching to assess changes in skin thickness and pliability. The soft tissue envelope is aggressively debulked over the sidewalls cephalad to the alar crease by resecting the SMAS layer. Once the SMAS and fibrofatty tissue has been freed from the overlying skin, it can then be carefully resected off the underlying cartilage and bone.

The soft tissue envelope can also be precisely debulked with a plucking technique using an Adson-Brown forceps. When extensive debulking has been performed, we find placement of suture-fixated soft tissue splint helpful in minimizing early postoperative edema. Prolonged edema of the soft tissue envelope has been reported to last 12 to 24 months. Meticulous intraoperative hemostasis, respect of tissue planes, use

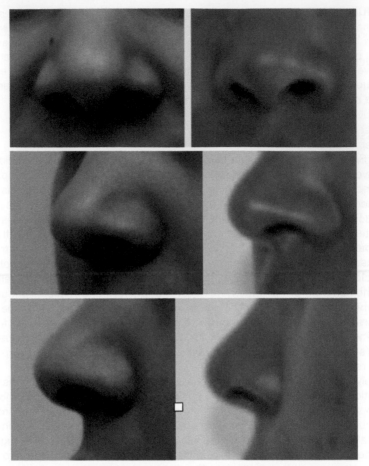

Fig. 6. Illustrative case. Patient with thick nasal skin, bulbous tip, wide nostrils, and flared alar. The nasal tip projection is adequate, therefore further tip projection is inappropriate in either achieving tip definition or alar flare reduction. The procedure was performed with endonasal approach, nasal skin envelope was selectively debulked over the tip and supratip area, suturing technique applied to reduce intradomal and interdomal angles, alar rim graft placed to reduce the degree of alar flare, and intrasill reduction to reduce alar base width.

of cool gauze compression throughout the case, together with extended postoperative splinting and taping is helpful in mitigating the edema. It is often necessary to serially inject steroid to further modulate the degree of subcutaneous scarring after aggressive skin debulking. Additionally, taping can also assist in allowing the swelling to resolve and the soft tissue to redrape. A series of triamcinolone injections is necessary to further modulate the degree of subcutaneous scarring.

ILLUSTRATIVE CASE

A patient of African descent with broad nasal tip, thick skin, wide alar base, and a flared alar with wide nostril is shown in **Fig. 6**. The patient was interested in rhinoplasty with ethnically congruent features.

DISCLOSURE

The author has nothing to disclose.

REFERENCES

1. Sofola IO, Boahene KDO. Rhinoplasty in the patient of African descent. Chapter 42. In: Papel ID, Frodel JL, Richard Holt G, et al, editors. Facial plastic and reconstructive surgery. 4th edition. New York: Thieme Medical; 2016. p. 518-30.
2. Walker-Smith GJ, Gale AG, Findlay JM. Eye movement strategies involved in face perception. Perception 1977;6:313–26.
3. Luria SM, Strauss MS. Comparison of eye movements over faces in photographic positives and negatives. Perception 1978;7(3):349–58.
4. Boahene KDO, Hilger PA. Alar rim grafting in rhinoplasty: indications, technique, and outcomes. Arch Facial Plast Surg 2009;11(5):285–9.
5. Kridel RW, Konior RJ, Shumrick KA, et al. Advances in nasal tip surgery: the lateral crural steal. Arch Otolaryngol Head Neck Surg 1989;115:1206–12.
6. Gassner HG, Mueller-Vogt U, Strutz J, et al. Nasal tip recontouring in primary rhinoplasty: the endonasal complete release approach. JAMA Facial Plast Surg 2013;15(1):11–6.
7. Kim MH, Choi JH, Kim MS, et al. An introduction to the septal extension graft. Arch Plast Surg 2014;41(1):29–34.
8. Toriumi DM. New concepts in nasal tip contouring. Arch Facial Plast Surg 2006; 8(3):156–85.

Moving?

Make sure your subscription moves with you!

To notify us of your new address, find your **Clinics Account Number** (located on your mailing label above your name), and contact customer service at:

Email: journalscustomerservice-usa@elsevier.com

800-654-2452 (subscribers in the U.S. & Canada)
314-447-8871 (subscribers outside of the U.S. & Canada)

Fax number: 314-447-8029

Elsevier Health Sciences Division
Subscription Customer Service
3251 Riverport Lane
Maryland Heights, MO 63043

ELSEVIER

Printed and bound by CPI Group (UK) Ltd, Croydon, CR0 4YY

03/10/2024

01040403-0007